Sarah Mang

Diffusion Simulation Based Tracking

Sarah Mang

Diffusion Simulation Based Tracking

And Optimized Gradient Encoding Schemes For Diffusion Magnetic Resonance Imaging

Südwestdeutscher Verlag für Hochschulschriften

Impressum/Imprint (nur für Deutschland/ only for Germany)
Bibliografische Information der Deutschen Nationalbibliothek: Die Deutsche Nationalbibliothek verzeichnet diese Publikation in der Deutschen Nationalbibliografie; detaillierte bibliografische Daten sind im Internet über http://dnb.d-nb.de abrufbar.

Alle in diesem Buch genannten Marken und Produktnamen unterliegen warenzeichen-, marken- oder patentrechtlichem Schutz bzw. sind Warenzeichen oder eingetragene Warenzeichen der jeweiligen Inhaber. Die Wiedergabe von Marken, Produktnamen, Gebrauchsnamen, Handelsnamen, Warenbezeichnungen u.s.w. in diesem Werk berechtigt auch ohne besondere Kennzeichnung nicht zu der Annahme, dass solche Namen im Sinne der Warenzeichen- und Markenschutzgesetzgebung als frei zu betrachten wären und daher von jedermann benutzt werden dürften.

Verlag: Südwestdeutscher Verlag für Hochschulschriften Aktiengesellschaft & Co. KG
Dudweiler Landstr. 99, 66123 Saarbrücken, Deutschland
Telefon +49 681 37 20 271-1, Telefax +49 681 37 20 271-0
Email: info@svh-verlag.de
Zugl.: Mannheim, Universität Mannheim, Diss., 2008

Herstellung in Deutschland:
Schaltungsdienst Lange o.H.G., Berlin
Books on Demand GmbH, Norderstedt
Reha GmbH, Saarbrücken
Amazon Distribution GmbH, Leipzig
ISBN: 978-3-8381-1381-4

Imprint (only for USA, GB)
Bibliographic information published by the Deutsche Nationalbibliothek: The Deutsche Nationalbibliothek lists this publication in the Deutsche Nationalbibliografie; detailed bibliographic data are available in the Internet at http://dnb.d-nb.de.

Any brand names and product names mentioned in this book are subject to trademark, brand or patent protection and are trademarks or registered trademarks of their respective holders. The use of brand names, product names, common names, trade names, product descriptions etc. even without a particular marking in this works is in no way to be construed to mean that such names may be regarded as unrestricted in respect of trademark and brand protection legislation and could thus be used by anyone.

Publisher: Südwestdeutscher Verlag für Hochschulschriften Aktiengesellschaft & Co. KG
Dudweiler Landstr. 99, 66123 Saarbrücken, Germany
Phone +49 681 37 20 271-1, Fax +49 681 37 20 271-0
Email: info@svh-verlag.de

Printed in the U.S.A.
Printed in the U.K. by (see last page)
ISBN: 978-3-8381-1381-4

Copyright © 2010 by the author and Südwestdeutscher Verlag für Hochschulschriften Aktiengesellschaft & Co. KG and licensors
All rights reserved. Saarbrücken 2010

Abstract

Diffusion tensor magnetic resonance imaging is the only non-invasive imaging technique that allows the discrimination of different matter types as well as the distinction of matter anatomy. Anatomy investigations are possible because the measured diffusion is stronger in parallel with boundaries, such as for example cell membranes. For the reconstruction of complicated anatomies, especially the pathways of neuronal brain fibers, fiber tracking methods were developed. The classical streamline tracking methods cannot handle voxels that contain multiple fiber orientations well. Examples for such multi-orientation voxels are voxels containing fiber crossing, fiber branching or kissing fibers. The directional heterogeneity in such voxels cannot be modeled with the simple second order diffusion tensor used for standard tracking, which can only model one dominating diffusion direction. I have developed a new diffusion simulation based fiber tracking method that uses time-of-arrival maps to reconstruct the tracts. This method is able to resolve a lot of problems of the commonly used streamline method. The reconstruction can also be performed on simulations that use more advanced diffusion models. A first simple example for such an extension of the diffusion simulation is discussed here.

To use more advanced diffusion models, such as the higher order tensor hierarchy, in a clinical environment the extensive measurement time required for the data acquisition for this model needs to be reduced. In my evaluations on gradient encoding schemes I investigated the required number of encoding directions and the distribution of the directions for higher order tensor estimations with several quality measures. I was able to show, that 21 directions are the minimal required number of encoding directions for the higher order tensor hierarchy model and that the paired off force minimizing gradient encoding scheme is the best all purpose scheme for diffusion evaluation with second or higher order tensor models.

Key words: DSBT, Fiber Tracking, Higher Order Tensors, Gradient Encoding Schemes

For a color version of the figures please refer to the online version of this text at http://madoc.bib.uni-mannheim.de/madoc/volltexte/2008/1913/.

Zusammenfassung

Diffusionstensor Magnetresonanz Bildgebung ist das einzige nicht-invasive Bildgebungsverfahren, das es erlaubt sowohl verschiedene Gewebearten zu unterscheiden als auch auf die Gewebeanatomie zu schließen. Rückschlüsse auf die Anatomie sind möglich, da die gemessene Diffusion stärker parallel zu begrenzenden Strukturen, wie zum Beispiel Zellmembranen, verläuft. Um komplizierte Anatomien, ins besondere Nervenbahnen im Gehirn, zu rekonstruieren wurden verschiedene Rekonstruktionsmethoden (so genannte „Fiber Tracking"-Verfahren) entwickelt. Die klassischen „Streamline"-Rekonstruktionsmethoden können Voxel mit mehreren Faserorientierungen (zum Beispiel Faserkreuzungen oder -verzweigungen) schlecht handhaben. Die in diesen Voxeln vorliegende

Heterogenität der Faserrichtungen kann nicht durch das einfach Tensormodell zweiter Ordnung, das von Standardrekonstruktionsverfahren benutzt wird, beschrieben werden, da es maximal eine dominante Diffusionsrichtung adäquat beschreiben kann. Ich habe eine neue diffusionssimulationsbasierte Methode zur Rekonstruktion von Nervenbahnen entwickelt, die Fasern unter der Verwendung von so genannten"Time-of-Arrival Maps" rekonstruiert. Diese Methode ist in der Lage einige Probleme der gebräuchlichen „Streamline"-Verfahren zu lösen. Außerdem kann dieses Rekonstruktionsverfahren auf beliebigen Diffusionssimulationen, also auch auf solchen, die kompliziertere Diffusionsmodelle verwenden, aufgesetzt werden. Ein erster Ansatz, eine solche weiterentwickelte Diffusionssimulation zu definieren, wird hier diskutiert.

Um kompliziertere Diffusionsmodelle, wie zum Beispiel Tensoren höherer Ordnung, in einem klinischen Kontext zu verwenden, muss die extrem lange Messzeit für die benötigten Daten reduziert werden. In meiner Betrachtung von Gradientenkodierschemata habe ich die benötigte Anzahl von Gradientenrichtungen und deren Verteilung mit verschiedenen Qualitätskriterien untersucht. Ich konnte zeigen, dass 21 Richtungen die minimal benötigte Anzahl an Richtungen für das Tensorhierarchie-Model sind und dass die paarwise Kräfteminimierung zwischen den Gradientenrichtungen die beste allgemeine Verteilung für die Auswertung von Tensoren jeder Ordnung liefert.

Schlüsselbegriffe: DSBT, Faserrekonstruktion, Tensoren höherer Ordnung, Gradientenschemata

Die Abbildungen in diesem Text in Farbe finden Sie in der digitalen Version unter http://madoc.bib.uni-mannheim.de/madoc/volltexte/2008/1913/.

Acknowledgments

A lot of people supported me during my work on this thesis. They did not only offer moral support but also valuable discussions and helped me find my way in the previously unknown world of neuroscience and MR. Thank you all for your help. I would also like to thank all the people, who helped with the actual writing of this thesis. This part of a project is always underestimated. During my work I was lucky enough to get to know many people, who are fascinated by neuroscience and MR. They taught me a lot and keep on rekindling my fascination with this topic. Thanks for that.

I would like to especially thank my supervisors Dr. Daniel Gembris and Prof. Dr. Reinhard Männer for their support and mentoring of this work. Dr. Daniel Gembris introduced me to MRI and did ignite my enthusiasm for DTI and fiber tracking. Lively discussions with him helped to clarify my ideas and concepts. Prof. Dr. Reinhard Männer was always very supportive and a calming influence in the institute.

Wolf Blecher, Markus Gipp and Felix Bootz gave the word 'group' a new meaning. I am forever grateful to them and all other members of the MR-technology group and the whole ICM for their support and ideas.

I am very grateful to Dr. Dimitrij Logashenko and Prof. Dr. Gabriel Wittum of the Steinbeis Research Center 936, Oelbronn-Duerrn, Germany, who supported my work with their expertise in diffusion simulation. The cooperation with them was full of interesting discussions, new ideas and will hopefully continue in the future.

Prof. Dr. Wolfgang Grodd and all people from the section of experimental magnetic resonance of the CNS took me in and made me welcome in the final phase of this project. I am very grateful for this, and appreciate their support more than I can say. Special thanks go to Prof. Dr. Uwe Klose and Dr. Michael Erb, who had always time to answer my questions and discuss new ideas. Prof. Dr. Uwe Klose did especially help me see my work in a more critical light.

I would also like to thank Dr. Chunlei Liu, Prof. Dr. Michael Moseley and Prof. Dr. Gary Glover for inviting me to Stanford. The opportunity to work in their lab was invaluable. All people at the Lucas Center made me feel welcome and showed me how bigger labs work. This experience and the numerous discussions helped me see my work and DTI in general in a new light. I am very grateful for that.

A special thank you goes to my family for supporting me during this demanding time.

Financial Support

This work was supported by Landesstiftung Baden-Würthemberg (Az.: 21-655.023/-Gembris and Az. Landesstiftung: 1.1611.0_).

My stay at Stanford University was supported by the Deutscher Akademischer Austausch Dienst (DAAD) with a Doktorandenstipendium (315 D/07/42989).

Contents

1. **Introduction**   1
   - 1.1. Motivation   1
   - 1.2. Outline   2
   - 1.3. Original Contributions   3
2. **Magnetic Resonance Imaging**   5
   - 2.1. The Magnetic Resonance Phenomenon   5
   - 2.2. Image Acquisition   7
   - 2.3. Imaging Contrasts   9
   - 2.4. Imaging Sequences   11
     - 2.4.1. Spin Echo Sequence   11
     - 2.4.2. Gradient Echo Sequence   13
     - 2.4.3. Echo Planar Imaging   13
   - 2.5. Imaging Quality   14
     - 2.5.1. Signal-To-Noise Ratio   15
     - 2.5.2. Partial Volume Effect   17
3. **Diffusion Weighted Imaging**   18
   - 3.1. The Anatomy Of Brain Connectivity - An Overview   18
   - 3.2. Diffusion Basics   20
   - 3.3. **k**-Space Diffusion Imaging   21
   - 3.4. **q**-Space Imaging   24
4. **Interpreting The Measured Diffusion**   26
   - 4.1. A Simple Interpretation Method   26
   - 4.2. The Diffusion Tensor   28
     - 4.2.1. Tensor Derived Diffusion Indices   31
     - 4.2.2. Tensor Visualization   34
   - 4.3. Recent Developments In Diffusion Evaluation   35
     - 4.3.1. Characterizing Diffusion With Spherical Harmonic Decomposition   36
     - 4.3.2. Multi-Tensor Approach   37
     - 4.3.3. Generalized Diffusion Tensor Imaging   38
5. **Gradient Encoding Schemes**   46
   - 5.1. Polyhedral Encoding Schemes   47

5.2.	Analytical Schemes	49
5.3.	Numerically Optimized Encoding Schemes	50
	5.3.1. Minimum Force Approach	50
	5.3.2. Minimal Condition Number Algorithm	52

6. Determining The Quality Of Encoding Schemes — 53

6.1.	The Evaluated GES	53
6.2.	Known Indices	55
	6.2.1. Total Variance	55
	6.2.2. Relative Encoding Advantage Factor	55
	6.2.3. The Condition Number Of The Estimation Matrix	56
	6.2.4. Guaranteed Anisotropic Sensitivity	56
6.3.	Total Variance Of The Second Order Tensor Estimation	57
6.4.	Classification By Condition Number For Higher Order Tensor Models	57
6.5.	Spread Of Directions	65
6.6.	Classification By Diffusion Index Estimation Quality	74
6.7.	Evaluation Of The Signal Representation	79
6.8.	Summary And Discussion Of The GES Evaluations	89

7. Fiber Tracking — 92

7.1.	Established Tracking Methods	93
	7.1.1. Streamline Tracking	93
	7.1.2. Front Propagating Methods	96
	7.1.3. Probabilistic Tracking	98

8. Diffusion Simulation Based Tracking — 101

8.1.	The Basic Algorithm	101
8.2.	The Simulation	102
	8.2.1. Initialization Of The Concentration Peak	102
	8.2.2. Implementation	104
8.3.	The TOA Map	106
8.4.	The Gradient Descend	110
8.5.	Problems With The Single Simulation Approach	112
8.6.	Successive Simulations	115
	8.6.1. Known Problems	117
8.7.	Tracking Acceleration	119
	8.7.1. Subgrid Resolution	119
	8.7.2. The Similarity Tract Termination Criterion	120
	8.7.3. Global Smoothness Tract Termination	122
	8.7.4. Look-Up-Table	123
	8.7.5. Propagator Approach	124
8.8.	Implementation	125
8.9.	Tracking Results	126
	8.9.1. Branching	128

8.9.2.	Orthogonal Crossing	130
8.9.3.	Straight Crossing	132
8.9.4.	Curve Crossing and Kissing	133
8.9.5.	Spiral	135
8.9.6.	Conclusion from the Comparison	135
8.9.7.	Discussions	136

9. Summary And Outlook   139

   9.1. Summary   139
      9.1.1. Higher Order Tensor Models   139
      9.1.2. Gradient Encoding Schemes   139
      9.1.3. Fibertracking   140
   9.2. Open Questions   142
      9.2.1. Higher Order Tensor Models   142
      9.2.2. Gradient Encoding Schemes   142
      9.2.3. Fibertracking   142

A. Tables With Results From GES-Evaluation   144

B. DTI-Studio Evaluation Parameters   149

C. Input Tensors For Simulations   151
   C.1. Second Order Tensors   151
   C.2. HOT Hierarchy Tensors   151

D. The Relationship Between The ADC Glyph And The Reynold Tensor Glyph   153

E. List of Figures   154

F. List of Tables   161

Abbreviations   163

Original Publications   165

Bibliography   167

1. Introduction

1.1. Motivation

Diffusion weighted (magnetic resonance) imaging is able to measure diffusion inside of a subject. The relevant molecular movement here is a random displacement of molecules relative to each other (Brownian motion). Opposed to the commonly known concentration driven diffusion this movement does not depend on a concentration gradient and is therefore also termed self-diffusion. The molecules are magnetically labeled prior to the image acquisition, depending on their position and the direction the diffusion is to be investigated in. At the time of image acquisition the position of the molecules has changed due to self-diffusion processes. The resulting local signal change is used to determine the amount of self-diffusion. The self-diffusion usually follows the path of least resistance, therefore it is faster parallel to barriers, such as cell membranes, than perpendicular to them. This phenomenon allows to non-invasively gather information on the structure of the subject matter from the acquired images. If several images are acquired (at least 6 diffusion weighted ones and 1 without diffusion weighting), the self-diffusion process can be modeled in 3D, for example with a second order diffusion tensor. From the 3D tensor important information can be extracted, such as the principal diffusion direction or the anisotropy of the local diffusion. This allows not only a distinction of matter types, for example gray and white matter in the brain, but also the distinction of coherent structures of one matter type, for example different neuronal fiber bundles with different orientations in the brain white matter. This structural information cannot be acquired with other non-invasive imaging modalities, which enhances the importance of diffusion weighted imaging for in vivo studies, for example on humans.

The resolution of diffusion weighted images is relatively coarse, in the order of millimeters, for the distinction of neuronal fibers, which have a diameter in the order of micrometers. The low resolution allows multiple fiber orientations inside of a measured voxel. This will cause problems for the standard second order tensor diffusion model, that is only able to model a single fiber orientation per voxel. Recently more advanced diffusion models have been proposed to overcome this limitation. These models require a larger number of diffusion encoding directions. I investigated the number of directions that is required for the evaluation of higher order tensor diffusion models and the optimal arrangement of these directions (see chapter 5).

Fiber tracking is a technique to reconstruct fiber bundles in 3D from the measured diffusion information. Most common techniques are line propagating techniques, which

1. Introduction

reconstruct the path of a fiber bundle step-by-step, following the principal diffusion direction. These methods have difficulties reconstructing the fiber pathways in voxels which contain more than one fiber orientation because they are based on the voxel wise evaluated second order tensor model that cannot adequately represent the diffusion in such heterogeneous voxels. To overcome the limitations of this tracking method I developed a front propagating fiber tracking technique that allows the reconstruction of crossing, branching and curving fibers (see chapter 7). This method is able to resolve a lot of problems of the commonly used streamline methods by considering a neighborhood of voxels in the reconstruction of the tract.

1.2. Outline

In chapter 2, the basics of magnetic resonance imaging are explained. First, the physical phenomena that are the basis for this technique are presented before the basics of magnetic resonance image acquisition are discussed in short. The image contrasts that are used to distinguish different matter types, are introduced before the most common imaging sequences are presented. A measure for imaging quality, the signal-to-noise ratio is presented before the partial voluming effect that is especially important in the context of diffusion tensor imaging is explained.

Chapter 3 starts with a short introduction to brain anatomy. The basics of diffusion are presented, before different diffusion weighting imaging methods are explored.

Different diffusion models can be fit to the signal in a set of diffusion weighted images. These models, derived scalar values and corresponding visualizations are presented and discussed in chapter 4. The most common diffusion model is the second order diffusion tensor which is presented in detail in 4.2. I explored the possibilities for the use of higher order tensor models for practical application, therefore the two known higher order tensor models are also presented and discussed in more detail (see 4.3.3).

In the course of my exploration of higher order tensor models, I investigated the influence of the gradient encoding schemes on the higher order tensor estimation. The discussions of higher order tensor models in literature (see for example [57, 73]) use large numbers of gradient encoding directions which require a prolonged data acquisition. I investigated how the number of required data acquisitions can be reduced to allow the use of these models in practical applications. Different families of gradient encoding schemes are presented in chapter 5. An attempt of determining the quality of the individual encoding schemes was made in 6. For this evaluation different encoding schemes were compared, using different quality measures known from literature and developed by myself.

In chapter 7 methods of fiber tracking, that are used to reconstruct neuronal fiber pathways in the brain white matter are presented. My diffusion simulation based tracking (DSBT) method, which uses time-of-arrival (TOA) maps, is introduced in chapter 8. This tracking method is based on the simulation of a diffusion process that is governed by the calculated diffusion tensors and propagates a diffusion front over the data set. The reconstruction follows the gradient on the so propagated fronts toward the simulation origin, allowing fiber branching to be handled automatically. This is one of the major advantages of this approach over more classical tracking methods. Another major advantage of DSBT is that the tract reconstruction can be based on any kind of diffusion simulation and is therefore not directly dependent on the second order diffusion tensor. If a more advanced diffusion model can be used in the simulation to generate more accurate diffusion fronts, the DSBT reconstruction based on these results will return more accurate fiber tracts. The method can therefore easily be extended to more advanced diffusion models, as long as a diffusion simulation can be computed with this model. This extension of DSBT and one possible alternative simulation are discussed in section 8.9.7.

In the last chapter, I will summarize my findings and present questions that are still open.

1.3. Original Contributions

In my investigations my main focus was on two subjects:

1. **The development of a new diffusion simulation based fiber tracking algorithm that uses time-of-arrival maps.** This technique consists of three major steps: the simulation of diffusion, the construction of a time-of-arrival map from the simulation results and the actual tract reconstruction on this map [Mang05, Mang05a, Mang05b, Mang06, Gembris07a]. It is able to continue tracking in regions of fiber crossing or branching, which contain more than one fiber direction [Mang06, Gembris07a]. The heterogeneity in these multi-directional voxels presents a problem for commonly used streamline tracking methods, which will return false reconstructions or aborted tracts. The algorithm is also able to reconstruct curving tracts that cannot be reconstructed by the streamline technique. A comparison of the results of my algorithm with streamline reconstructions is given in section 8.9 to illustrate the advantages of the here presented new tracking method.

2. **The qualitative assessment of diffusion weighting gradient encoding schemes for higher order tensor estimations.** After reducing the minimal required number of encoding directions for the higher order hierarchy estimation to 21 directions (see section 4.3.3.2), I evaluated how the directions should be distributed over the unit sphere, so as not to bias the tensor estimation [Mang07, Mang07a]. I discovered that for the minimal number of encoding directions at least two diffusion weighting factors (greater zero) are required to successfully estimate the tensor (see section 4.3.3.2). I could show that several quality measures for gradient encoding schemes for second order tensor evaluations are either not fit to determine the quality the higher order tensor estimation or are in general not well suited for determining the quality of gradient encoding schemes (see chapter 6). Several other quality measures did allow a classification of gradient encoding schemes for

1. Introduction

different tensor models. The most promising classification method in the here presented investigation was a new classification method I proposed in section 6.7, the *evaluation of the signal accuracy*. This method allows a clear distinction between (most) gradient encoding schemes. It was shown that icosahedral and paired off force-minimizing distributions of encoding directions perform best. The paired off force-minimization can construct encoding schemes with an arbitrary number of directions, opposed to the icosahedral encoding schemes that can only be constructed for certain fixed numbers of directions. This force-minimizing gradient encoding scheme is therefore considered the best general purpose scheme in my investigation.

2. Magnetic Resonance Imaging

Magnetic resonance imaging (MRI) is in general a tomographic imaging technique which is able to acquire detailed images of body tissue. MRI requires no ionizing radiation (for example x-ray) and is therefore less risky for the patient's health. During a MRI scan often a series of parallel slice images of the measured subject is acquired. These 2D images can be used to generate a 3D dataset in post-processing. Volumetric image acquisition methods were proposed to acquire whole 3D data sets, see for example [62].

Volumetric imaging is not yet commonly used for the measurement of diffusion, which is the focus of this work. This image acquisition method is therefore not further discussed here.

One of the advantages of MRI is the ability to image soft tissues and the metabolic processes therein. This is in general not possible with alternative imaging techniques such as for example computer tomography.

To measure subject matter with MRI one requires radio frequency pulses, imaging gradients and a strong static magnetic fields. The technique can be used to image specific molecules in a subject. In clinical MRI the focus is mainly on the protons of hydrogen (H) atoms. Approximately two thirds of the human body consist of water (H_2O) providing high, almost equally distributed hydrogen nuclei density and therefore good signal strength over the whole body. To achieve good imaging quality, a stable and homogeneous static magnetic field is required. Superconducting electromagnets with additional 'shimming' to improve the homogeneity are used to generate a magnetic field suitable for MR-scanning. In the context of MRI, 'shimming' is the name for all procedures used prior to the actual imaging process to correct for macroscopic inhomogeneities in the static magnetic field. In clinical applications field strengths of 1.5 Tesla and 3 Tesla are common for the applied static magnetic field.

In this chapter some basic terms and methods are introduced that will be used throughout the rest of the text. The magnetic resonance phenomenon that is the foundation of MRI is explained first. Then, the commonly used basic imaging sequences are introduced before the different imaging contrasts are explained. At the end of this chapter the signal-to-noise ratio and the partial voluming effects are presented.

2.1. The Magnetic Resonance Phenomenon

Here the magnetic resonance phenomenon is explained using a classical representation which ignores interactions of the protons with their surroundings. The effect of the

2. Magnetic Resonance Imaging

gradients on the protons is explained on a single proton example. Each individual proton can only produce a minuscule signal but the sum of all protons in the sample is able to generate significant signal.

A proton has two features that are important in context of MRI (see Fig.2.1). One is its angular momentum, that is the rotation of the proton around its own axis which is illustrated as stippled line in Fig.2.1. The other is its magnetic moment caused by the proton's rotating positive electric charge, resulting in its behavior as little magnet (see Fig.2.1(b)).

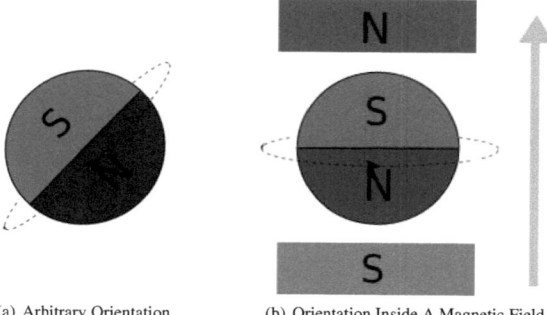

(a) Arbitrary Orientation (b) Orientation Inside A Magnetic Field

Figure 2.1.: *The two properties of a proton that are important for MRI are illustrated.*

In an environment without an external magnetic field the axis of a proton is arbitrarily orientated in space (Fig.2.1(a)). On entering the strong static magnetic field of the scanner (B_0) the proton will align itself with this field as illustrated in Fig.2.1(b). This state is the state of equilibrium of the nuclear magnetization under the influence of B_0. The rotating magnetization of a proton is further on simply called 'spin'.

Due to change in the magnetic field the spin can leave its equilibrium and the axis of the proton will be oriented at an angle to the axis of B_0. Its angular momentum causes the proton to precess around the axis of B_0, if it is not in its state of equilibrium. The frequency of the precession ω_0 is dependent on the applied magnetic field.

$$\omega_0 = \gamma |B_0|, \tag{2.1}$$

where ω_0 is the so called resonance or Larmor frequency (usually given in Mega Hertz (MHz)), γ is the so-called gyromagnetic ratio and $|B_0|$ is the magnitude of the static magnetic field commonly measured in Tesla (T). The Larmor frequency of hydrogen is 42.58MHz at 1T.

The phase of the spin determines its position on the circle that is described by its precession around the axis of B_0. The spin is usually depicted as an arrow in the direction of the rotation axis of the spin. By convention the Z-axis of the measurement coordinate system corresponds to the main axis of B_0.

2.2. Image Acquisition

If an additional electromagnetic field at a frequency of ω_0 is applied perpendicular to the static magnetic field B_0 for a short time. The spins will leave their equilibrium. This process is called 'excitation'. The electromagnetic field of short duration that is used for the excitation is also called radio frequency (RF) pulse. If the duration of the RF pulse is correctly adjusted, the spin is rotated in a 90 degree angle to B_0, it 'flips' (see Fig.2.2). The result of excitation is also referred to as transversal magnetization. After excitation the spin will return to its equilibrium under the influence of B_0. This process is called 'relaxation' and allows different matter types to have a distinct imaging contrast allowing their separation. Relaxation will be discussed in more detail in the section on imaging contrasts 2.3.

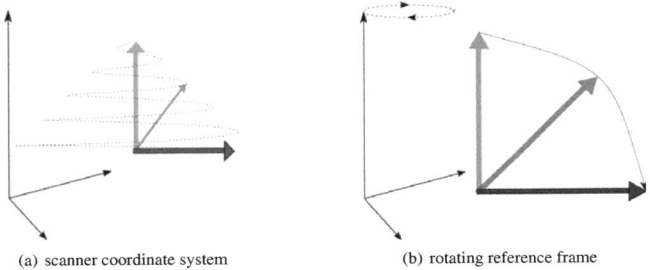

(a) scanner coordinate system   (b) rotating reference frame

Figure 2.2.: *The net magnetization flips into the XY-plane.*

In the measurement or scanner coordinate system the spin precesses around the axis of B_0 at Larmor frequency as soon as it leaves its equilibrium. The excited spin will therefore describe a circle in the XY-plane. During the transition between equilibrium and transversal magnetization (during the 'flip') the precession will cause the spin to describe a spiral around the axis of B_0 as illustrated in Fig.2.2(a). To facilitate the description of the behavior of the spin, the 'rotating reference frame' is introduced. It is assumed that the coordinate system rotates around the Z-axis (the axis of B_0) at Larmor frequency (see Fig.2.2(b)). This allows for the spin vector in this rotating coordinate system to appear stationary.

2.2. Image Acquisition

The magnetic resonance signal can be described as

$$S(\mathbf{k}) = \int \rho(\mathbf{r}) exp(i2\pi \mathbf{k}\mathbf{r}) d\mathbf{r}, \qquad (2.2)$$

with i the imaginary unit ($i^2 = -1$), $\mathbf{k} = (2\pi)^{-1}\gamma \mathbf{G}t$, $\mathbf{r}$ the particle position, $\rho(\mathbf{r})$ the particle concentration, $\mathbf{G}$ the ideally rectangular gradient, t the gradient duration and γ

2. Magnetic Resonance Imaging

the gyromagnetic ratio that corresponds to the Larmor frequency ($\gamma = 42.58 MHz/T^{-1}$). **k**-space is usually traversed in time. It is also possible to traverse it in gradient magnitude [17], but this is not done in common image acquisition. The Cartesian image $I(\mathbf{r})$ is the Fourier-transform of the signal $S(\mathbf{k})$,

$$I(\mathbf{r}) \approx \rho(\mathbf{r}) = \int S(\mathbf{k}) exp(-i2\pi \mathbf{k}\mathbf{r})d\mathbf{k}. \tag{2.3}$$

k-space is, in other words, conjugate to the Cartesian image space.

Slice Selection And Spatial Coding

In common applications the MRI signals are acquired as 2D images. To be able to generate a 2D image the signal needs to be dependent on the position of the spins that generate it. This is achieved by application of additional linear changing magnetic fields in the signal acquisition.

As long as B_0 is homogeneous the spins all have the same Larmor frequency and will consequently all be excited by the same RF pulse. The application of a monotone linear changing magnetic field, also called gradient **G** (**G** = G**g**; with G the strength of the magnetic gradient field and **g** its direction), which is independent of the stronger B_0, causes the spins to have individual local Larmor frequencies given by

$$\omega_0(\mathbf{r}) = \gamma B(\mathbf{r}) = \gamma(|B_0| + G(\mathbf{r})), \tag{2.4}$$

where $G(\mathbf{r})$ stands for the strength of the gradient magnetic field at position **r** which is a spin coordinate. This enables a selective excitation with a tailored RF pulse because the Larmor frequency is proportional to the total strength of the applied magnetic field $B(\mathbf{r})$ which is dependent on **r**.

The applied gradient fields (ideally) only influence the magnetization in Z-direction as illustrated in Fig.2.3 where the Z-direction corresponds to the axis of the green tube that stands for the magnet producing the static magnetic field B_0. The magnetization vectors (red) all point along the Z-direction independent on the gradient that was applied. The strength of the magnetization illustrated in the length of the magnetization vectors varies depending on the gradient direction.

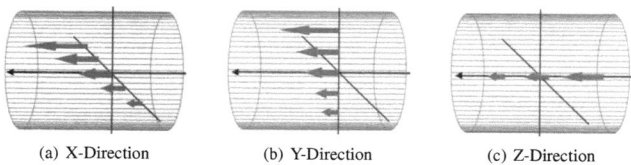

(a) X-Direction   (b) Y-Direction   (c) Z-Direction

Figure 2.3.: *The effect of linear gradient on the static magnetic field B_0. Illustration adopted from [67].*

2.3. Imaging Contrasts

To excite the protons in a certain slice a gradient in Z-direction is applied (Fig.2.3(c)) so that the Larmor frequency of the spins is dependent on their position along the Z-axis. The RF pulse used for the excitation is tailored to the specific Larmor frequency of the spins in a specific slice. The width of the slice is determined by the bandwidth of the RF pulse and the gradient field strength. A narrower bandwidth or a stronger gradient causes thinner slices if the other parameter (gradient strength or RF bandwidth respectively) is fixed.

To be able to distinguish between the signal of individual voxels in the slice, two more gradients are needed. The change in Y-direction is phase encoded and in X-direction the frequency codes changes. After an RF pulse has excited the spins a gradient in Y-direction is used to create a linear development in the Larmor frequency. In the following it is assumed to descend from the top of the magnet. This leads to a phase shift in the individual spins, which codes the position in Y-direction. When the gradient is turned off, the phase shift persists. To differentiate pixels in X-direction, a gradient is applied in this direction. This will cause the strength of the magnetic field to increase from one side to the other. Here a left to right slope in the magnetic field is assumed. The protons on the left precess slower then the ones on the right.

When the signal $S(\mathbf{k})$ is measured for a given slice, the gradients generate a frequency spectrum, high frequencies correspond to the right side of the acquired image, low frequencies to the left side. In $\mathbf{k}$-space the horizontal, k_x, is the frequency direction and the vertical, k_y is the phase direction. Each line corresponds to a single signal acquisition, for each phase gradient a new line is created. The line at $k_y = 0$ corresponds to the measurement without phase encoding. With a Fourier transform (FT) along the frequency direction, the position in X-direction in image space is decoded. To decode the phase information, the measurement needs to be repeated several times (once for each step in Y-direction). Then a second FT can be preformed in phase direction decoding the Cartesian pixel coordinates. The reconstruction of a complete 2D slice is called 2D FT reconstruction.

2.3. Imaging Contrasts

MR-measurements are sensitive to specific molecular properties of matter in the magnetic field of the scanner, such as for example relaxation times. This makes the non-invasive distinction of different matter types possible, which is one of the primary advantages of MR.

There are two kinds of relaxation that give different imaging contrasts:

- **the T_1 relaxation time** is the time needed by the excited spins to return to their state of equilibrium.

- **the T_2 relaxation time** is the time during which the MR signal decays due to interactions between nuclei.

2. Magnetic Resonance Imaging

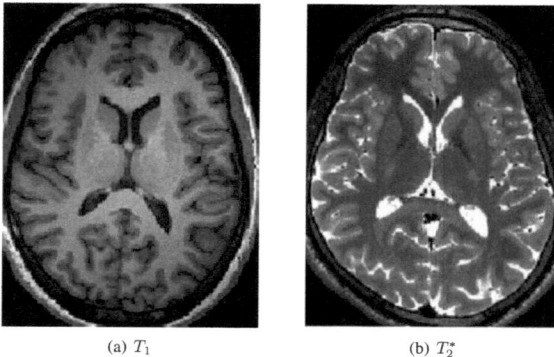

(a) T_1 (b) T_2^*

Figure 2.4.: *Example images for the two main imaging contrasts.*

With these two attributes, different types of matter can be distinguished without use of contrast agents. In Fig.2.4 examples for both imaging contrasts are shown.

The strength of T_1 contrast depends on the time between two excitations (TR). Not all spins have enough time to realign themselves with B_0 when the TR is shorter than the typical T_1 time in the sample. The measured signal is maximal for spins that are aligned with B_0 before the next excitation (light regions in Fig.2.4(a)). The further away a spin is from its state of equilibrium at the time of refocusing, the lower the signal (darker parts of Fig.2.4(a)). When TR is long, most spins align themselves with B_0 before the next excitation, the T_1 contrast is consequently negligible.

The T_2 contrast depends on the time between the excitation pulse and signal (echo) generation, known as (spin) echo time (TE). After the excitation the spins will dephase. This loss of phase coherence is matter dependent and caused by interactions of neighboring spins in an ideal homogeneous magnetic field. The T_2 effect is boosted by inhomogeneities of the magnetic field. Examples for causes of inhomogeneity are susceptibility or chemical shift phenomena. Susceptibility gives the extent of magnetization of subject matter on entering a magnetic field. The chemical shift gives the difference in magnetic energy levels depending on the molecule environment. The total signal decay, the regular T_2 effect and dephasing caused by gradients, is labeled T_2^*. The more dephased the spins of the nuclei in a voxel are, the weaker their signals in the measurement. The longer TE, the more time the spins of the nuclei have to dephase. Matter with short T_2 time will therefore return a low signal when the TE is long (darker parts of the Fig.2.4(b)). The shorter the TE, the weaker the T_2 contrast.

2.4. Imaging Sequences

In general all MRI sequences consist of 3 parts:

1. **excitation**
2. **spin rephasing**
3. **echo generation**

An echo is an electromagnetic resonance signal emitted from the spins after excitation. The main difference between the imaging sequences is the way the echoes are produced by application of specific RF-pulses and magnetic field gradients. A few important sequences are briefly discussed in the following sections. The presented sequences acquire the **k**-space data line by line on a Cartesian grid. It is possible to acquire the signal following some other acquisition scheme, for example spirals [34]. These techniques will not be discussed further here.

2.4.1. Spin Echo Sequence

One of the most common imaging sequences is the spin echo sequence. Here the signal is generated by a spin echo (more accurately the Hahn spin echo [38, 39]). The diagram in Fig.2.5 shows the different stages of the spins during an echo generation. Important times in the sequence are given in the top row to facilitate comparison with the gradient and RF pulse application shown in Fig.2.6 which shows the timing of the image acquisition.

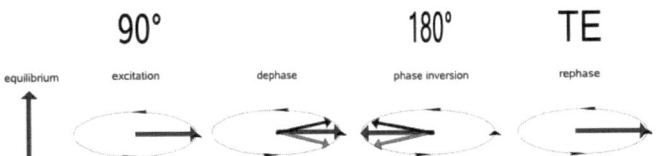

Figure 2.5.: *The stages of the magnetization in the image acquisition.*

The first stage in Fig.2.5 shows the spins before excitation in the state of equilibrium, aligned with B_0. The second stage is the excitation. The spins in one slice are excited by the application of a 90 degree RF pulse, flipping the spins into the transversal XY-plane, perpendicular to B_0. In the third stage, immediately after the excitation, the spins begin to dephase due to T_2/T_2^* relaxation and the imaging gradients [14]. The individual spins (vectors in Fig.2.5) are not aligned anymore. They precess around B_0 with different frequencies. The higher the frequency (faster rotation), the darker the color. After half of the TE has passed, a 180 degree RF pulse is applied. This causes the spins to rotate 180 degree about the X-axis. The phase order of the spins is thereby reversed, the one with the lowest frequency will be first the highest last. Only the phase, not the frequency,

2. Magnetic Resonance Imaging

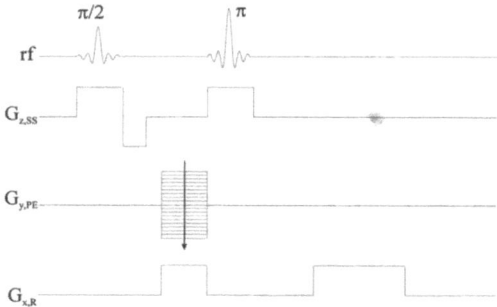

Figure 2.6.: *A diagram depicting a simple spin echo sequence (image adopted from [36]).*

of the spin is affected by the second pulse. Therefore, the spins will realign themselves (rephase) at the echo time (TE) to form the echo.

The **k**-space is traversed line by line in this sequence. Each line in this simple spin echo sequence requires one excitation. This means multiple excitations or 'shots' are needed to cover the whole **k**-space. The spin echo sequence and all sequences that need multiple excitations to traverse **k**-space are referred to as multi-shot methods.

The sequence diagram of a simple spin echo sequence is given in Fig.2.6. First, the phase encoding gradient amplitude $G_{y,PE}$ is used to target the line in **k**-space that is to be acquired. The multiple lines in $G_{y,PE}$ (see Fig.2.6) and the downward arrow indicate that the phase encoding gradient is changed stepwise sequentially from its most positive to its most negative amplitude. One step for each line in **k**-space. The amplitude of the frequency encoding gradient $G_{x,R}$ is constant, to travel along the line in **k**-space from sample point to sample point. The signal is acquired at different equally spaced time points.

The spin echo sequence is not sensitive to static field inhomogeneity that could cause image distortion. A disadvantage is the relatively long TE, which renders the sequence more susceptible to motion artifacts. Such motion artifacts can result from any kind of patient movement for example slight turning of the head, breathing or cardiac motion.

The TR gives the time required for one signal acquisition in a slice. There is some idle time for the imaging hardware (TR-TE) during a signal acquisition cycle. To increase the efficiency of the measurement other slices can be excited and measured during this idle time. This technique is called multi-slice imaging. Another way to improve measurement time efficiency if a slice needs to be measured repeatedly, is the use of multiple echoes. A train of rapidly applied 180 degree RF pulses serves to generate repetitive signal echoes, one for each pulse in the train. The most common multi-echo sequence is the turbo spin echo (TSE) sequence.

2.4. Imaging Sequences

2.4.2. Gradient Echo Sequence

This sequence uses only the gradients and no RF pulse to generate an echo [93]. After the excitation pulse the read out gradient G_R is applied causing the spins to dephase (see discussion of T_2/T_2^* in 2.3). Then the gradient's polarization is inverted to reverse this effect and rephase the spins to generate an echo. The sequence is given in Fig.2.7 where G_{ss} is the slice selection gradient and G_{PE} is the phase encoding gradient. By toggling

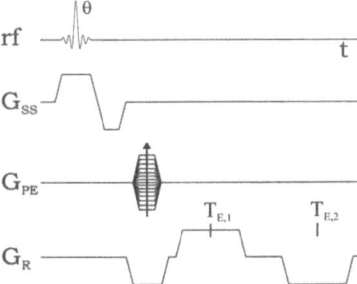

Figure 2.7.: *A diagram of the gradient echo sequence (image adopted from [36]).*

G_R repeatedly multiple echoes can be generated. The behavior of the spins is similar to the one during the spin echo sequence illustrated in Fig.2.5.

The measurement time is reduced compared to the spin echo sequence, because no 180 degree RF pulse is required in this sequence and the excitation pulse can have less than 90 degree. If the excitation pulse is reduced (less than 90 degree) the transversal magnetization is incomplete because the proton magnetization does not flip into the XY-plane but precesses at an angle that depends on the excitation pulse relative to the Z-axis. The signal will therefore be less than the one the perfect 90 degree RF pulse could generate. The reduced flip angle will result in reduced relaxation time, the proton magnetization will return faster to their state of equilibrium. The next excitation can, therefore, be applied sooner reducing the measurement time. The reduction of the total measurement time reduces the possibility of motion artifacts. To render the sequence even more efficient multiple echoes can be generated by toggling the frequency coding gradient several times. This sequence is similar to the spin echo sequence, a multi-shot method, which travels through **k**-space one line at a time.

2.4.3. Echo Planar Imaging

Echo Planar Imaging (EPI) is a rapid pulsed gradient echo MRI sequence. The technique collects complete 2D images (slices) with Cartesian **k**-space coverage. In its simplest form only one excitation RF pulse is used for the signal acquisition (single shot). Other

2. Magnetic Resonance Imaging

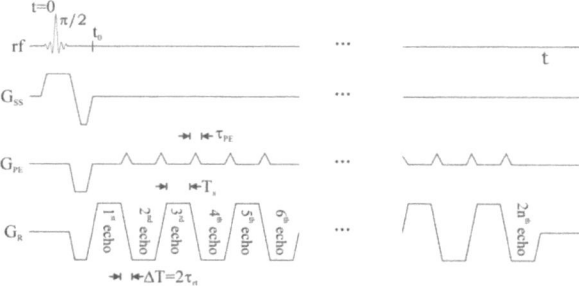

Figure 2.8.: *EPI sequence timing diagram with an echo train (image adopted from [36])*.

imaging techniques read out one line per excitation only and are consequently considerably slower then EPI. This rapid sequence creates echoes, similar to the gradient echo sequence, by toggling the frequency coding gradient periodically as illustrated in the sequence diagram in Fig.2.8. Each echo contains the readout for a whole line in **k**-space. The line that is to be read is determined by the phase encoding gradient strength (G_{PE}). The first line to be read is targeted with the first application of the phase encoding gradient. When the signal for this line is acquired the line is changed by a short phase encoding gradient pulse (a blib).

EPI images have good imaging quality if no local magnetic field gradients are present in the investigated subject matter. In brain investigations this would correspond to the center of the brain. Local gradients as, for example, caused by the paranasal sinuses in the human head, will cause geometric and signal distortions in the image [36]. The local gradients add to the applied gradient field and will cause a faulty position reconstruction for the distorted signal.

2.5. Imaging Quality

The images acquired with MRI are often compromised by either random noise, systematic measurement errors or other artifacts that can stem from numerous sources [93, 36]. Some examples are hardware related, such as inhomogeneous magnetic fields or not well calibrated imaging coils, or sequence related, for example violations of the Nyquist-Shannon sampling theorem[1] or non-optimal measurement parameters. Other artifacts are caused by image processing or patient movement during the scan.

In the following section the signal-to-noise ratio (2.5.1) is presented as measure for image quality. Then the partial-voluming effect (PVE) (2.5.2), is discussed in more

---

[1]"Exact reconstruction of a continuous-time baseband signal from its samples is possible, if the signal is bandlimited and the sampling frequency is greater than twice the signal bandwidth." http://www.en.wikipedia.org

2.5. Imaging Quality

detail because it is of special interest in the context of diffusion evaluations (see chapter 4).

2.5.1. Signal-To-Noise Ratio

Each measured signal S consists of the true MR signal S_{true} and random noise η,

$$S = S_{true} + \eta. \tag{2.5}$$

The signal-to-noise ratio (SNR) describes the relation between true signal and random noise in an MRI experiment. It is more specifically defined as the relation between the true signal and the standard deviation of the noise:

$$SNR = \frac{S_{true}}{\sigma(\eta)}. \tag{2.6}$$

SNR is a widely used measure for image quality (the higher, the better). The SNR can depend on a lot of different measurement and subject parameters.

$$SNR \propto \left\{ \rho \delta_v \delta_\phi \delta_s \sqrt{N_v} \sqrt{N_\phi} \sqrt{N_{rep} \frac{1}{\sqrt{\Delta v_{samp}}}} \omega_0 \right\} f_M f_T, \tag{2.7}$$

with ρ the nuclei density and $\delta_v \delta_\phi \delta_s$ the voxel volume. N_v is the number of frequency coding steps, N_ϕ is the number of phase coding steps and N_{rep} is the number of repeated acquisitions of the image volume. Δv_{samp} is the sampling bandwidth, which gives the range of frequencies for sampling the signal. ω_0 is the Larmor frequency. f_M is a function, depending on the imaging sequence parameters such as, for example, flip-angle, pulse sequence, TE and TR. f_T is a function that depends on the properties of the investigated tissue, for example, T^1 and T^2. Imaging Hardware and subject motion can further influence the SNR [93]. Here the focus is on the dependence of the SNR on the imaging resolution. The general diffusion analysis (see chapter 4) and especially fiber tracking (see chapter 7) requires high resolution images thereby lending the SNR dependence on the voxel volume special importance. An increased image resolution can be achieved by reducing the field of view for a given number of voxels or by increasing the number of voxels for a given field of view. Both methods decrease the individual voxel volume. The dependence of the SNR on the voxel volume can be easily explained. Random noise is independent of the measurement and therefore of the voxel volume. Opposed to that the signal depends on the number of spins inside a voxel which will decrease proportional to the voxel volume. The SNR will therefore decrease proportional to the intensity of the true signal.

Averaging over multiple repeated (N_{rep}) acquisitions is common practice [36] for the compensation of the loss in SNR caused by the reduction of the individual voxel's volume. For more efficient storage the measured signals are added directly, saving a considerable amount of data storage space.

$$S_{av} = \frac{1}{N_{rep}} \sum_{i=1}^{N_{rep}} S_i, \tag{2.8}$$

2. Magnetic Resonance Imaging

S_{av} is the signal averaged over N_{rep} measurements. S_i is the signal in the i-th acquisition. If the mean signal $\overline{S}$ over a homogeneous region is averaged, the following conclusion holds [36]:

$$\overline{S_{av}} = \frac{1}{N_{rep}} \sum_{i=1}^{N_{rep}} \overline{S_i} = \frac{1}{N_{rep}}(N_{rep} S_{true}) = S_{true}. \tag{2.9}$$

The Gaussian normal distributed ($N(0, \sigma)$) noise in each of the N_{rep} measurements is statistically independent for the individual measurements. Therefore the noise distribution's averaged variance $\sigma_{av}^2(\eta)$ adds in quadrature to S_{av},

$$var(S_{av}) \equiv \sigma_{av}^2(\eta) = \frac{1}{N_{rep}^2}(N_{rep}\sigma_{av}^2(\eta)) = \frac{1}{N_{rep}}(\sigma_{av}^2(\eta)). \tag{2.10}$$

It follows that

$$\sigma_{av}(\eta) = \frac{\sigma(\eta)}{\sqrt{N_{rep}}}. \tag{2.11}$$

The SNR of the averaged image is therefore

$$SNR = \frac{\overline{S_{av}}}{\sigma_{av}(\eta)} = \sqrt{N_{rep}} \frac{S_{true}}{\sigma(\eta)}. \tag{2.12}$$

In other words, if the noise in the measurement is uncorrelated from one acquisition to the next, the SNR improves as the square root of the number of repetitions. To avoid errors introduced during averaging, the individual images should be realigned. Realignment matches corresponding regions so that the voxels that are averaged (ideally) correspond to the same region.

The systematic noise which is not statistically independent for each acquisition will not reduce in the same way. Examples for systematic noise are ghosting and drifts. If the systematic noise is greater than the random noise, averaging does not improve the SNR according to (2.12). The gain of additional acquisitions in this case does in general not warrant for the increase in measurement time.

An approximative estimation of the SNR for an actual image is simple: first, the mean value of a small region of interest placed inside the most homogeneous region with high signal intensity in the measured subject is computed ($\overline{S}$). Second, the standard deviation in the largest possible region outside the object (σ_{out}), i.e. in the background which only contains noise, is calculated. The SNR is then given by

$$SNR = \frac{\overline{S}}{\sigma_{out}}. \tag{2.13}$$

This estimation of the noise has the problem that the noise in the background has a mean of zero. The measured signal is usually a magnitude image $|S|$. The parts of the noise in the background that would be negative are, therefore, in the magnitude image also positive. It follows that the mean value in the selected background region is larger zero and that the corresponding standard deviation of the noise σ_{out} is lower than it would

2.5. Imaging Quality

be if estimated in a large homogeneous region with high signal (for example in a water phantom) where the true mean corresponds to the true signal value instead of zero. The estimation of σ_{out} inside, for example, the brain is not possible because of the multiple matter contrasts that allow no homogeneous region large enough for the estimation.

2.5.2. Partial Volume Effect

Partial volume effect (PVE) is a name for all effects caused by the size of a voxel. PVE especially describes the loss of contrast between two or more adjacent tissues, caused by lack of image resolution. Low spatial resolution results in heterogeneous voxels that contain multiple matter types. The signal in such a voxel will represent the signal of the different matter types, weighted according to their occurrence in the voxel.

It is assumed that the investigated sample contains two separable kinds of matter, A and B, and S_A, respectively S_B, is the signal of a voxel (size Δx) containing only matter A, respectively B. If a voxel contains both kinds of matter, with a the fraction of the voxel occupied by tissue A, then the total signal S for this voxel is computed as follows

$$S = a\Delta x S_A + (1-a)\Delta x S_B. \tag{2.14}$$

The signal in such a heterogeneous voxel results from averaging, which diminishes the

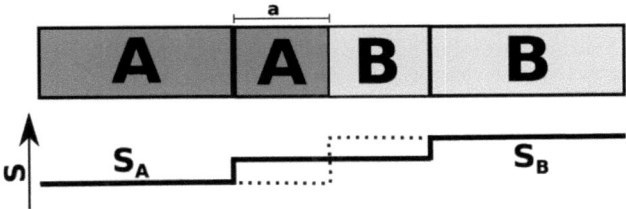

Figure 2.9.: *An example for PVE in a voxel with two kinds of matter.*

contrast on the border between two matter types. This is illustrated in Fig.2.9. In the top row the voxels are given. They contain matter A with lower signal and matter B with higher signal. The signal amplitude is shown as a dark line in the bottom row. The signal of the center voxel containing both matter types is the average of S_A and S_B. The ideal signal that would not diminish the contrast between the matter types is given as dotted line.

3. Diffusion Weighted Imaging

When measuring diffusion with MRI techniques the focus is commonly on the Brownian motion (also known as self-diffusion) of water or more exact of the hydrogen in the water molecule. The self-diffusion inside subject matter is in general not free, but hindered or restricted by anatomy. Membranes for example hinder self-diffusion by troubling the passage of molecules. Other structures, for example bones, do not let any molecule pass and restrict the self-diffusion. This influence of the anatomy on self-diffusion allows for the inference of the anatomy from the measured self-diffusion information. The technique used for the measurement of self-diffusion is called diffusion weighted imaging (DWI) and measures the amount of self-diffusion in a given direction. To do that, the molecules are magnetically labeled before the signal is acquired. The magnetization from this labeling is reversed prior to the echo generation. Stationary molecules will return the full signal whereas molecular motion reduces the signal in DWI images.

The only diffusion process of interest in this work is the self-diffusion process. The term diffusion is therefore used synonymously to self-diffusion in the following text, except in the section on diffusion basics (3.2).

The focus in this work is on the investigation of brain connectivity, this is therefore the only part of the human anatomy that is presented in the first section of this chapter. Then the basics of diffusion are introduced before different diffusion imaging methods are discussed. The focus is mainly on the differences in interpretation of the measured results. It has to be kept in mind that different imaging techniques measure different quantities and these can in general not be compared directly.

3.1. The Anatomy Of Brain Connectivity - An Overview

The cortex is the 2-5 mm thick outermost layer of the brain. It is folded to allow a larger surface on a relatively small volume. The furrows of this folding are called sulci and the ridges are known as gyri as illustrated in Fig.3.1. The whole brain is divided in the middle, forming two (connected) hemispheres. The cortex consists of gray matter (GM), which is mainly responsible for computation in the brain. GM consists to a large part of neurons (see Fig.3.2(a)), but may also contain some axons, synapses, dendrites, and glial cells.

The white brain matter (WM) which is enclosed by the GM consists mainly of axons. The axons can be viewed as the wiring between the GM's computational units. WM axons are often well isolated by myelin sheets that are tightly wrapped around the axon

3.1. The Anatomy Of Brain Connectivity - An Overview

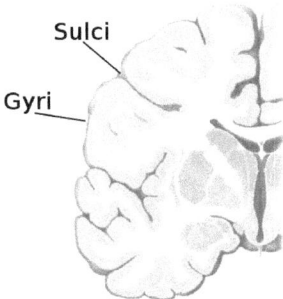

Figure 3.1.: *Coronal cut through the brain. The gray matter is the darker outermost region of the brain. It encloses the white matter. The brain surface is folded producing sulci (grooves) and gyri (elevations). Image adapted from [82].*

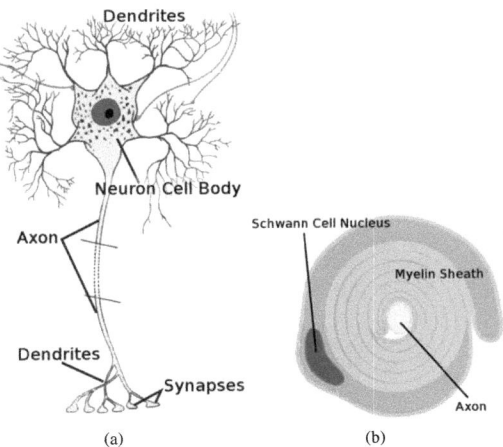

Figure 3.2.: *The anatomy of a neuron is illustrated in (a). The axon of a neuron is isolated by a myelin sheath that is wound tightly around the fiber as illustrated in a cut through the axon in (b). The illustrations were adapted from [89]*

to improve the information transfer (see Fig.3.2(b)). The myelin is the cause of the white coloring that gave the WM its name. Myelinated axons in the brain have usually a length of approximately 1-10 cm and 1-10 μm in diameter. They are often organized in bundles of 2 mm up to 1 cm thickness. The course of the highly organized and well isolated WM fiber bundles can be investigated with DWI.

The whole brain is suffused with liquid, the so called cerebrospinal fluid. This fluid has numerous responsibilities, for example the transport of neurotransmitters and the protection of the brain from increased blood pressure. The brain also contains several other structures, such as for example the thalamus or the hypothalamus. These important and complicated structures are not discussed in this basic introduction.

3.2. Diffusion Basics

Diffusion abides to laws similar to heat. It can therefore be described with Fick's first law, which is similar to the law of heat conduction,

$$J = -D\nabla C. \tag{3.1}$$

J is the particle flux, D is the diffusion coefficient and ∇C is the particle concentration gradient, $\frac{\partial C}{\partial \mathbf{r}}$ with $\mathbf{r}$ a coordinate in 3D [22]. According to this equation the particle flux is proportional to the diffusion coefficient. This is the classical description of diffusion. The continuity theorem,

$$\frac{\partial C}{\partial t} = -\frac{\partial J}{\partial \mathbf{r}}, \tag{3.2}$$

that describes the conservation of mass over time t can be used to derive the diffusion equation, also known as Fick's second law [71]

$$\frac{\partial C}{\partial t} = \nabla(D\nabla C). \tag{3.3}$$

This differential equation gives the time and space dependent change in concentration opposed to Fick's first law which is not time dependent.

Self-diffusion is defined as the random movement of molecules in matter. This motion can be described with the self-correlation function $P_s(\mathbf{r}|\mathbf{r}', t)$ [16], which gives the chance that a molecule will have moved from $\mathbf{r}$ to $\mathbf{r}'$ after time t. The total probability of finding a particle at position $\mathbf{r}'$ at time t is given by

$$\rho(\mathbf{r}', t) = \int \rho(\mathbf{r}, 0) P_s(\mathbf{r}|\mathbf{r}', t) d\mathbf{r}. \tag{3.4}$$

$\rho(\mathbf{r}, 0)$ is here the initial particle concentration in $\mathbf{r}$ at $t = 0$. There is no net concentration gradient for the self diffusion processes that are (usually) measured with diffusion weighted MR imaging techniques. A description of the diffusion process abiding the principle of Fick's law is still possible substituting the concentration function C with the concentration probability $\rho(\mathbf{r}', t)$. Now Fick's first law can be rephrased in terms of P_s because the spatial derivatives in this law refer to the particle position $\mathbf{r}'$ after the diffusion time t.

$$J = -D\nabla P_s, \tag{3.5}$$

with the initial condition

$$P_s(\mathbf{r}|\mathbf{r}', 0) = \delta(\mathbf{r}' - \mathbf{r}). \tag{3.6}$$

The continuity theorem is also applicable to this problem because the total conditional probability is conserved [16]. Combining (3.2) with (3.5) results in a differential equation similar to Fick's second law (3.3)

$$\frac{\partial P_s}{\partial t} = \nabla(D\nabla P_s). \tag{3.7}$$

It is assumed that the diffusion described by the diffusion coefficient D is unrestricted (free). The average diffusion distance of molecules can, therefore, be quantified with Einstein's equation $\sigma = \sqrt{2Dt}$. If the diffusion is free, the distribution of the molecules can be described with a Gaussian function

$$\frac{1}{\sigma\sqrt{2\pi}}e^{-x^2/2\sigma^2}, \tag{3.8}$$

where x is the molecule location. Free diffusion is, therefore, also termed 'Gaussian diffusion'

By substituting σ in (3.8) with Einstein's equation and the molecule location with the displacement vector $\mathbf{r}' - \mathbf{r}$, the self-correlation function P_s can be given by

$$P_s(\mathbf{r}|\mathbf{r}', t) = (4\pi Dt)^{-3/2} exp\left(-(\mathbf{r}' - \mathbf{r})^2/4Dt\right). \tag{3.9}$$

If the described diffusion is free $P_s \mapsto 0$ as $\mathbf{r}' \mapsto \infty$. The randomness of the particle motion in self-diffusion is reflected by the fact that P_s is only dependent on $\mathbf{r}'$ but not on $\mathbf{r}$.

With the displacement vector $\mathbf{R} = \mathbf{r}' - \mathbf{r}$ (3.4) can be rephrased in terms of $\overline{P_s}$ which is also referred to as '(average) propagator'.

$$\overline{P_s}(\mathbf{R}, t) = \int \rho(\mathbf{r}, 0) P_s(\mathbf{r}|\mathbf{r} + \mathbf{R}, t) d\mathbf{r}. \tag{3.10}$$

$P_s(\mathbf{r}|\mathbf{r} + \mathbf{R}, t)$ is independent of $\mathbf{r}$ in free diffusion. In this case the propagator $\overline{P_s}$ is common to all protons in the averaged sample, therefore $\overline{P_s}(\mathbf{R}, t) = P_s(\mathbf{R}, t)$. (3.9) can be rephrased with the propagator formalism from (3.10) as

$$P_s(\mathbf{R}, t) = (4\pi Dt)^{-3/2} exp\left(-\mathbf{R}^2/4Dt\right). \tag{3.11}$$

3.3. k-Space Diffusion Imaging

To measure diffusion the MR signal needs to be sensitized to the movement of molecules caused by diffusion. This can be achieved by application of two additional gradients in

3. Diffusion Weighted Imaging

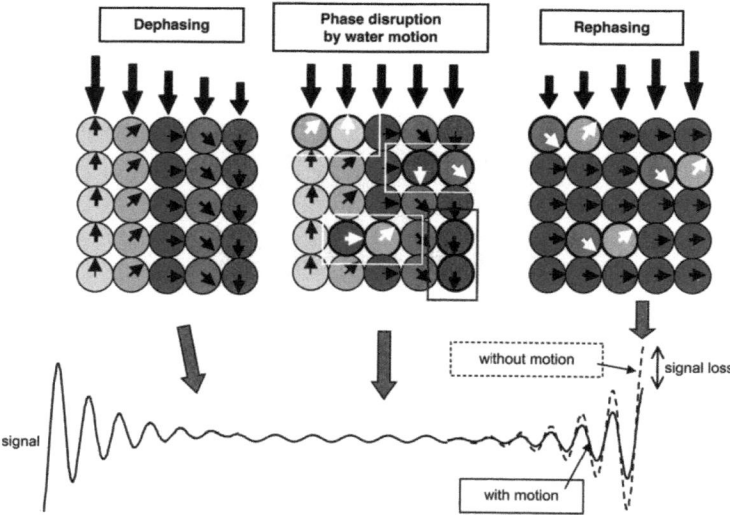

Figure 3.3.: *The effect of diffusion wheighting on the signal. The illustration was addopted from [67].*

the imaging sequence as illustrated in Fig.3.3. The gradients are depicted as large black arrows in Fig.3.3. The first gradient magnetically labels the protons according to their position. This additional gradient affects the phase of the spins which is now dependent on the spin position ('Dephasing' in Fig.3.3, the phase is color coded). The effect of this label is reversed before the images are acquired by a second gradient which is the inverse of the first one. On stationary molecules the application of the two diffusion weighting gradients has no effect (purple in 'Rephaseing' in Fig.3.3) but for molecules that have moved the inversion of the magnetic labeling will not be perfect. The phase shift caused by the first diffusion weighting gradient will not be (completely) reversed. This results in a reduction of the acquired MR signal. The effect of diffusion is therefore coded in the signal reduction in the diffusion weighted image compared to the signal without diffusion weighting.

The diffusion weighted image is sensitive only for diffusion along the axis of the applied diffusion weighting gradient (left-right in Fig.3.3; yellow boxes). Movement in other directions (green box) is not detected.

A simple kind of DWI uses the pulsed gradient echo sequence (PGES) [86] to measure diffusion in **k**-space. This sequence is based on the spin echo sequence presented in section 2.4.1. The diagram in Fig.3.3 illustrates the timing of the additional diffu-

3.3. k-Space Diffusion Imaging

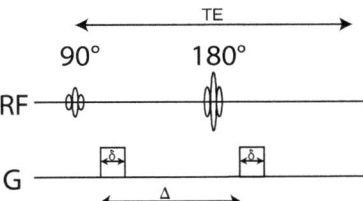

Figure 3.4.: *Pulsed gradient echo sequence for diffusion weighted imaging.*

sion weighting gradients. First, the spins which are aligned with the B_0 gradient field are flipped into the XY-plane by a 90 degree radio frequency pulse. Now, a diffusion weighting gradient is applied in a specified direction to label the individual spins with phase shifts according to their position. At $t = TE/2$ the phase of the individual spins is inverted with a 180 degree radio frequency pulse before a second diffusion weighting gradient, inverse to the first one, is applied to reverse the position dependent labeling.

The signal for a voxel is always a superposition of all the spins in this voxel (with additional cross-contamination from neighboring voxel signals which is ignored in this description of the principle). There is no way to distinguish the signal from individual spins. The individual paths of the molecules are of no consequence, only the total phase difference at different time points is measured. Therefore, the measured diffusion is an ensemble-average of the self-diffusion processes in each voxel. The measured signal is consequently symmetric. There is no difference between the measured signal in direction **g** and the signal measured in the opposite direction (−**g**) because the net displacement is the same. This allows for a reduction in required measurements since only one of the two directions on an axis needs to be measured.

The relation between the measurements with ($S_\mathbf{g}$) and without (S_0) diffusion weighting will give the diffusion coefficient in the direction of the diffusion weighting (Stejskal-Tanner equation):

$$S_\mathbf{g} = S_0 exp(-bD_\mathbf{g}) \qquad (3.12)$$
$$D_\mathbf{g} = -\frac{1}{b}ln(S_\mathbf{g}/S_0),$$

g is the normalized direction of the diffusion weighting gradient. b represents the influence the gradient parameters have on the measurement, in other words the strength of the diffusion weighting. For an ideal rectangular gradient in the standard pulsed gradient echo sequence (illustrated in Fig.3.3) b is given by

$$b = \gamma^2 G^2 \delta^2 (\Delta - \delta/3) \qquad (3.13)$$

with γ the gyromagnetic ratio, G the diffusion gradient magnitude, δ the duration of the gradient and Δ the time span from the application of one gradient to the next. $D_\mathbf{g}$ in

3. Diffusion Weighted Imaging

(3.12) is the measured diffusion coefficient. The diffusion coefficient gives the amount of diffusion in the direction of the diffusion weighting gradient **g**. Only the apparent effect of diffusion but not the true diffusion coefficient is measured, because the diffusion investigated here is not free but hindered. D is therefore also referred to as 'apparent diffusion coefficient'. In this theoretical discussion of the measurement techniques it is assumed that the measurements are not affected by noise. The effects of noise in the data is discussed in chapters 2 and 4.

3.4. q-Space Imaging

q-Space Imaging (QSI) uses the **k**-space DWI gradient setup as illustrated in Fig.3.3 to generate a new imaging contrast that corresponds to molecular motion caused by diffusion. In QSI the diffusion weighting gradients need to be infinitesimal short, so the diffusion during the gradient application δ can be neglected. In other words, $\delta \ll \Delta$ is a necessary condition for QSI [17]. This was no requirement for **k**-space DWI.

QSI is similar to the introduced **k**-space DWI dependent on two gradient pulses defined by their magnitude G, duration δ and separation Δ. These properties clearly define the start and end point of the measured molecule movement over a well defined time Δ, as long as the movement during gradient application is negligible. Opposed to **k** in **k**-space imaging **q** is not used to spatially code the MR signal.

QSI measures the net phase shift directly which describes the measured diffusion. The signal is defined as

$$S(\mathbf{q}) = \int \overline{P_s}(\mathbf{R}, \Delta) exp(i2\pi \mathbf{q}\mathbf{R}) d\mathbf{R}. \tag{3.14}$$

$\overline{P_s}$ was defined in (3.10) and i again the imaginary unit. $\mathbf{R} = \mathbf{r}' - \mathbf{r}$ is the net displacement which is in QSI independent of the starting ($\mathbf{r}$) and endpoint ($\mathbf{r}'$). **q** is defined as $\mathbf{q} = (2\pi)^{-1}\gamma\delta\mathbf{G}$. The QSI signal is symmetric. The equation $S(\mathbf{q}) = S(-\mathbf{q})$ holds, if the only difference between both signals is the sign of the orientation **g** of the diffusion weighting gradient **G**.

q determines the diffusion weighting in the measurement. It contains information on the gradient strength G and duration δ similar to the diffusion weighting factor b in **k**-space DWI (see (3.13)). In addition **q** also contains the direction of the applied gradient **g** because $\mathbf{G} = G\mathbf{g}$. An additional multiplication with the gradient direction as in DWI (see (3.12)) is therefore not necessary.

The QSI signal as defined in (3.14) is not spatially dependent and is therefore averaged over the whole sample. When this pure QSI is combined with **k**-space imaging techniques it can be resolved for the individual voxels. Usually the PGES sequence from **k**-space imaging is used to implement a spatial resolution.

$$S(\mathbf{k}, \mathbf{q}) = \int \rho(\mathbf{r}) S(\mathbf{q}) exp(i2\pi \mathbf{k}\mathbf{r}) d\mathbf{r}, \tag{3.15}$$

with $S(\mathbf{q})$ as defined in (3.14) and the other variables as introduced in (2.2). Further on, I will use the term QSI for this combined imaging technique.

3.4. q-Space Imaging

QSI is able to measure dynamic displacement whereas **k**-space DWI measures static displacement. Therefore, QSI needs, opposed to the ordinary (**k**-space) DWI interpretation which assumes Gaussian diffusion, not make any assumptions on the underlying diffusion model in the interpretation of the measurement. A technique that is independent of an underlying diffusion model is also termed 'model-free'. The restrictions on molecular movement by anatomy causes the average displacement distribution to deviate from the Gaussian form of free diffusion, rendering model-free methods advantageous. If the measured diffusion is free $\overline{P_s}$ is equal to P_s. In this case QSI is equal to **k**-space DWI.

QSI is able to find existing restrictions and barriers for the diffusion, characterize anatomical compartments and resolve multiple fiber orientations. It can assess separately the effects of change in diffusion time, orientation and length scale on the displacement distribution depending on the diffusion weighting parameters [7]. This imaging technique is therefore successfully used in the investigation of static materials [17]. For in vivo studies, especially on humans, there are some limitations. The required gradient field and pulse strength present problems for the scanners in clinical use today. This makes it impossible to meet the condition of infinitesimal short δ in actual measurements with PGSE sequences.

The development of the STEAM (stimulated echo acquisition mode) sequence [72] makes real QSI on standard scanners possible. This imaging sequence can not reduce δ, but is able to allow large Δ, so $\delta \ll \Delta$ is satisfied. A large Δ may allow spins to wander between voxels, which might cause blurring in the measurement. As previously discussed prolonged measurement time allows for more motion artifacts and therefore presents an additional problem for QSI acquisition. This imaging sequence is not yet commonly used in clinical application.

Another alternative uses constant twice-refocused balanced echoes in the image acquisition [90]. The use of constant gradients clearly violates the 'narrow-pulse' approximation that is the basis of QSI. The propagator measured in this approach does not measure the probability density function of spin displacement directly but only the corresponding center-of-mass propagator [90, 65], which can also be used to measure displacement without the assumption of a Gaussian molecule distribution.

4. Interpreting The Measured Diffusion

Further processing of the diffusion information is necessary to facilitate its interpretation. For this purpose several diffusion indices and diffusion models were proposed. In the first section of this chapter, the most basic model free interpretation method is discussed. Then, the standard diffusion model, the second order diffusion tensor, is introduced. Some of the commonly used scalar diffusion measures which can be derived from this second order tensor model are presented. The second order diffusion tensor model is based on the assumption of Gaussian diffusion with mono-exponential signal decay. This assumption is not necessarily valid for the measured diffusion since the measurement grid is very coarse (see for example [3]). The measured diffusion can therefore contain the actual diffusion information of several diffusion compartments (PVE), this may result in a measured diffusion that is non-Gaussian. More advanced evaluation techniques which address this problem are presented in the last section of this chapter.

4.1. A Simple Interpretation Method

The simplest way to characterize diffusion measured in DWI is based on the apparent diffusion coefficient (ADC). The ADC is estimated as follows,

$$ADC = -\frac{1}{b}ln(S_{\mathbf{g}}/S_0). \tag{4.1}$$

Here b is the diffusion weighting factor, S the diffusion weighted signal and S_0 the unweighted signal. This definition corresponds to the definition of the self-diffusion coefficient in (3.12). The ADC describes the apparent diffusion recognizing the fact that measured diffusion is not free but hindered by barriers such as for example cell membranes. The measured diffusion coefficient is therefore not a diffusion coefficient as known in physics but the effect from diffusion, which is hindered by membranes. If free diffusion is the only motion present in a homogeneous environment, i.e. the measurement is noise and artifact free, the ADC is equal to the self-diffusion coefficient in the direction corresponding to the diffusion weighting of S. If the diffusion is isotropic (equally strong in all directions), a scalar ADC is sufficient to describe the diffusion.

If diffusion is anisotropic (not of equal strength for all possible directions) one scalar ADC is not sufficient for the representation of this diffusion process. If a HARDI data set

4.1. A Simple Interpretation Method

with a large number of different diffusion encoding gradient directions is acquired, the ADC of the individual gradient directions can be used to evaluate the overall diffusion profile. The estimated profile gets more accurate with an increase in diffusion encoding gradient directions, due to the increased angular resolution of the signal sampling.

Visualization The measured ADC information is hard to comprehend without adequate visualization. An intuitive form of visualization is the so called ADC map. It associates the measured, scalar ADC value to each voxel and is usually visualized as intensity map. The ADC can be evaluated and visualized as intensity map for each dif-

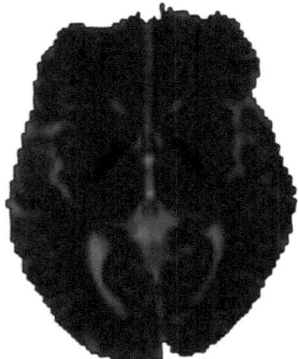

Figure 4.1.: *An example ADC intensity map.*

fusion encoding direction separately. More common is a map that codes the mean ADC as intensity value. In this map the information from the individual acquired directional images is combined.

This method gives a detailed representation of the measurements. It also gives an exact representation of the measured signal including the noise. This true representation of noisy data renders reproduction of the results difficult because of the randomness of the noise.

A 3D representation of the ADCs in each voxel is also possible. A three dimensional representation of the local diffusion information in a voxel is called glyph. The ADC glyph is a deformed sphere. The directions for which the ADC was computed (directions of the corresponding diffusion weighting gradients) are identified with points sampling a sphere. The radius of the sphere in each of the sampling points is set equal to the corresponding ADC. An example for a voxel containing a single fiber is given in Fig.4.2(a). It shows the typical peanut shape (For more on the shape of the ADC glyph and its relation to the Reynolds tensor glyph (introduced in section 4.2.2) see appendix D.).

4. Interpreting The Measured Diffusion

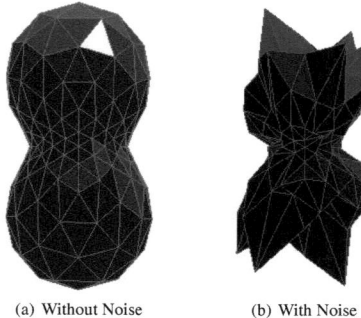

(a) Without Noise   (b) With Noise

Figure 4.2.: *ADC glyph for 81 gradient encoding directions.*

The ADC glyph in real data always is a corrupted representation of the underlying voxel micro-structure. The effect is illustrated in Fig.4.2, where a glyph without noise (Fig.4.2(a)) is given next to a glyph representing the same signal with noise (SNR = 10; Fig.4.2(b)).

4.2. The Diffusion Tensor

A more compact representation for the measured diffusion process is the second order 3x3 diffusion tensor. This symmetric positive definite tensor **D** contains only six independent components (see Fig.4.3). The diagonal elements of the tensor are related to the strength of the diffusion in the X-, Y- and Z-direction of the scanner coordinate system, respectively (see for example [2, 48]). The off-diagonal elements indicate the interdependence of the individual directions.

Therefore, the tensor can be computed from a minimum of one unweighted image and six diffusion weighed images for each voxel in the data set (see Fig.4.3). The use of several unweighted images and a larger number of diffusion weighting gradient directions will increase the estimation quality (as shown for example in [47] and my more extensive evaluations later on presented in chapter 5). A simple and explicit way to compute the diffusion tensor from seven measurements was described in [9]. The measurement of the required data for the tensor estimation is often referred to as diffusion tensor imaging (DTI).

The second order tensor is in literature (see for example [2, 92, 48]) defined so that the directional diffusion coefficient $D_\mathbf{g}$ is given by

$$D_\mathbf{g} = \mathbf{g}^T \mathbf{D} \mathbf{g}. \tag{4.2}$$

4.2. The Diffusion Tensor

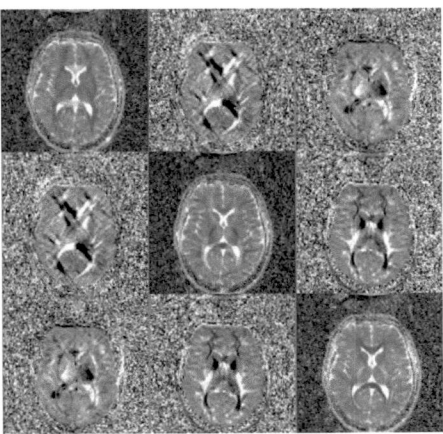

Figure 4.3.: *The symmetric tensor is illustrated. Each of the nine images gives the tensor elements, here visualized for a single slice in the data set. The off-diagonal images are mirrored on the diagonal. There are therefore only six different images (independent tensor elements). The signal in the diagonal tensor elements is stronger and less noisy than in the off-diagonal images.*

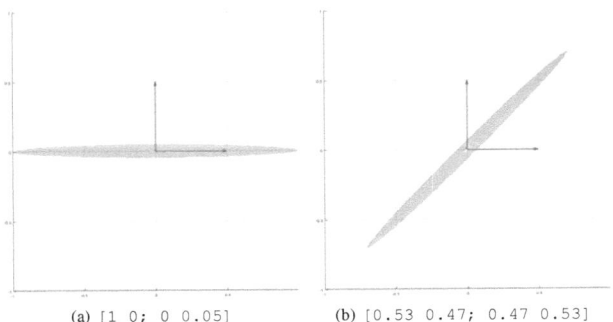

(a) [1 0; 0 0.05]   (b) [0.53 0.47; 0.47 0.53]

Figure 4.4.: *The off-diagonal elements give the tilt of the diffusion glyph. This is illustrated in two 2D examples. The tensor elements are given in the subtext of the plots.*

4. Interpreting The Measured Diffusion

This allows the extension of (3.12) for a second order diffusion tensor $\mathbf{D}$ to

$$S_g = S_0 exp(-b\mathbf{g}^T \mathbf{D} \mathbf{g}) \quad (4.3)$$

$$\Leftrightarrow ln\left(\frac{S_g}{S_0}\right) = -\sum_{\alpha=1}^{3}\sum_{\beta=1}^{3} b\mathbf{g}_\alpha \mathbf{g}_\beta \mathbf{D}_{\alpha\beta}. \quad (4.4)$$

Above $\mathbf{D}_{\alpha\beta}$ are the elements of the diffusion tensor, b is the diffusion weighting factor, S_0 is the unweighted signal, $\mathbf{g}$ the diffusion gradient direction vector. α and β are the element indices of the gradient vector $\mathbf{g}$ and diffusion tensor $\mathbf{D}$ that may take any Chartesian direction (x, y or z). S_g is the echo signal obtained for the applied diffusion gradient $\mathbf{g}$ with diffusion weighting b.

The tensor can be estimated by solving

$$\mathbf{BD} = \mathbf{Y} \quad (4.5)$$
$$\Leftrightarrow \mathbf{D} = \mathbf{B}^{-1}\mathbf{Y},$$

with $\mathbf{Y}$ a vector containing the logarithmic signal intensities $\overline{ADC} = ln(S_g/S_0)$ ($Y = \left[\overline{ADC}^1, \overline{ADC}^2 \ldots \overline{ADC}^{N_e}\right]^T$. $\mathbf{D}$ here is a vector containing the six independent second order diffusion tensor components. The effects the imaging gradients and the diffusion weighing gradient pulses have on the signal are embodied in the estimation matrix $\mathbf{B}$ whose elements corresponding to the gradient direction j ($j \in \{1,2,3\ldots N_e\}$, where N_e is the number of gradient encoding directions used in the estimation.) are defined as [63],

$$d^j = b\mathbf{g}_\alpha^j \mathbf{g}_\beta^j = b\left[\begin{array}{cccccc} g_{xx}^j & g_{yy}^j & g_{zz}^j & g_{xy}^j & g_{xz}^j & g_{yz}^j \end{array}\right]. \quad (4.6)$$

The complete matrix $\mathbf{B}$ has the form:

$$\mathbf{B} = \left[d^1, d^2, \ldots, d^{N_e}\right]^T. \quad (4.7)$$

The values on the diagonal of the diffusion tensor give the diffusion strength in the X-, Y- and Z-direction. The off-diagonal elements give the interdependence of the individual directions. This is illustrated in Fig.4.4. Where the same tensor shape is given in two orientations in the coordinate system. The off-diagonal elements determine the tilt of the tensor.

DTI is up till now only able to measure voxels with a side length larger than one millimeter on clinical scanners but single axons have a much smaller diameter of few micrometers. The coarseness of the DTI resolution allow that fibers with different orientations are contained in one voxel, a so called heterodirectional voxel [32]. This heterogeneity causes PVE. Each fiber will add to the signal intensity resulting in an averaged signal for a heterogeneous voxel. Under the assumption that there is no exchange between individual fiber bundles, the signal S is given by

$$S = \sum_{i=1}^{n} \alpha_i F_i. \quad (4.8)$$

4.2. The Diffusion Tensor

Here, n is the number of fiber bundles contained in a voxel, F_i is the signal produced by fiber i which is weighed according to its volume fraction α_i [3]. To reduce the PVE, one can increase image resolution at the expense of SNR. The reduction in SNR limits the increase in image resolution as well as the increase in measurement time. The measurement time increases exponentially with the increase in resolution. If the voxel length is halved in each direction the scan duration is $2^8 = (2^2)^3$ times prolonged.

The second order tensor is based on the assumption of homogeneous diffusion inside a voxel. This assumption allows for a maximum of one fiber orientation per voxel. Heterogeneous voxels presents a problem because the diffusion in this type of voxel cannot be adequately approximated by mono-exponential Gaussian diffusion (due to PVE).

4.2.1. Tensor Derived Diffusion Indices

From the second order diffusion tensor several useful scalar diffusion indices can be derived that characterize the diffusion inside a given voxel. The most commonly used indices are briefly presented in the following.

4.2.1.1. General Diffusion Indices

General diffusion indices characterize the diffusion processes inside of a voxel as a whole. The amount of diffusion is characterized but no directional dependence of the diffusion is explored. These indices can be computed without diagonalization of the diffusion tensor and can therefore be evaluated very fast.

One of the simplest indices is the trace tr of the diffusion tensor,

$$tr(\mathbf{D}) = \sum_{\alpha=1}^{3} \mathbf{D}_{\alpha\alpha}. \tag{4.9}$$

Here, $\mathbf{D}_{\alpha\alpha}$ are the elements on the diagonal of the diffusion tensor $\mathbf{D}$. The trace is rotationally invariant. In the context of DTI this means that the orientation of the fiber in relation to the diffusion weighting gradient direction set used in the acquisition is of no consequence. Since the diagonal elements give the diffusion strength in X-, Y- and Z-direction, these three gradient encoding directions are sufficient to compute the trace. If no more advanced evaluation is required, the number of DWI measurements can therefore be cut in half.

The mean diffusivity ($\bar{\mathbf{D}}$) is one of the oldest diffusion indices used in DTI. It is defined as the determinant of the diffusion tensor and therefore also rotationally invariant. A faster way of computation for this diffusion index is

$$\bar{\mathbf{D}} = \sum_{\alpha=1}^{3} \mathbf{D}_{\alpha\alpha}/3 = tr(\mathbf{D})/3, \tag{4.10}$$

which can also be computed from a minimum of three DWI images.

4. Interpreting The Measured Diffusion

4.2.1.2. Anisotropy

More detailed information on the diffusion inside of a voxel can be acquired with so called anisotropy indices. These indices describe the dominance of certain diffusion directions over others. The anisotropy information is dependent on the whole tensor. It is also dependent on the tensor orientation in the coordinate system given by the set of directions used in the DTI measurements and therefore called 'rotationally variant'. This dependence is discussed in more detail in my evaluation of gradient encoding schemes that will be presented in chapter 5. Anisotropy indices are a popular means for many disciplines, some examples are the investigation of (degenerating) neuronal disease, brain development or stroke. In the next paragraphs, the two most prominent anisotropy indices are presented in more detail.

Relative Anisotropy: The relative anisotropy (RA) is proportional to the standard deviation of the mean diffusivity from the individual eigenvalues:

$$RA = \frac{\sqrt{3}\sqrt{(\lambda_1 - \bar{D})^2 + (\lambda_2 - \bar{D})^2 + (\lambda_3 - \bar{D})^2}}{tr(\mathbf{D})}. \tag{4.11}$$

The λ stand for the three eigenvalues of the tensor $\mathbf{D}$. The three eigenvalues represent the magnitude of the diffusion in the direction of the corresponding eigenvectors. $\bar{D}$ stands for the mean diffusivity as previously defined in (4.10). RA can take values between 0 for fully isotropic voxels and $\sqrt{2}$ for highly anisotropic voxels.

Fractional Anisotropy: The fractional anisotropy (FA) is the most commonly used anisotropy index in clinical application. It is defined as

$$FA = \sqrt{\frac{3}{2} \frac{(\lambda_1 - \bar{D})^2 + (\lambda_2 - \bar{D})^2 + (\lambda_3 - \bar{D})^2}{\lambda_1^2 + \lambda_2^2 + \lambda_3^2}}. \tag{4.12}$$

λ and $\bar{D}$ are used as previously defined. It can take values from 0 (fully isotropic) to 1 (highly anisotropic), which is one of the reasons this index is preferable over others. Its interpretation is also slightly different from RA. It is a measure for the diffusion strength attributed to directional diffusion [6]. To speed up the computation, it can be computed without actually diagonalizing the estimated the tensor directly from the tensor elements [41]. It was also shown that the FA is more robust toward noise than RA [40]. The FA maps have a higher SNR than corresponding RA maps.

4.2.1.3. Directional Information in Scalar Maps

Often not only the scalar diffusion properties but also the principal direction of the diffusion is of interest in an investigation. The directional information facilitates for example the distinction of individual fiber pathways that lie close together but have different orientations. The primary eigenvector corresponds to the largest eigenvalue. It gives the

4.2. The Diffusion Tensor

principal diffusion direction that is assumed to correspond to the fiber orientation in this voxel. The information of a specific diffusion index can be combined with the directional information from the principal eigenvector. In a combined image the diffusion index is usually coded in the intensity and the color coding usually represents the three components of the primary eigenvector in RGB. This visualization method is illustrated on the example of a FA map in Fig.4.5. A prominent advantage of combining the FA with color-

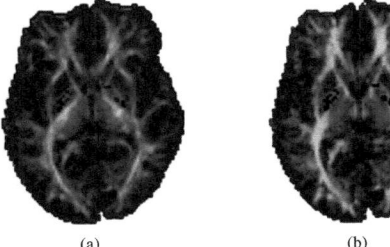

(a) (b)

Figure 4.5.: *In this figure the advantage of color coding the directionality of the measured diffusion information in a scalar diffusion index is illustrated on the example of FA maps. The FA is a scalar value that is usually visualized as intensity map in gray scale, as shown in (a). In (b) the FA is coded in the intensity values and the main diffusion direction is used for color coding. This allows a more detailed investigation of the diffusion.*

coded diffusion direction can be observed in the center of the example images in Fig.4.5 (see enlarged details in Fig.4.6). Here, the gray scale image does not allow the distinction between the fiber populations of different orientation. Especially the transition from the top-down (green) fibers of the inferior fronto-occipital tract and the front-back (blue) fibers of the internal capsule is not distinguishable.

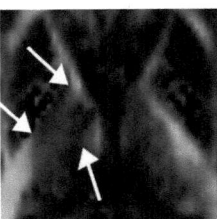

Figure 4.6.: *The importance of color coding is illustrated on an enlargement of the centers of the images in Fig.4.5. The transition, for example, of the green and blue fibers in the center cannot be distinguished from the gray scale image. Some of these regions that are not distinguishable without color-coding are indicated with white arrows.*

4.2.2. Tensor Visualization

To facilitate the interpretation of the diffusion tensor data, it is often useful to visualize it in 3D. A commonly used method to visualize a second order 3x3 diffusion tensor $\mathbf{D}$ is the *Lamé ellipsoid*. This glyph's orientation corresponds to the principal diffusion direction. The three radii are given by the three eigenvalues λ_i of the tensor $\mathbf{D}$ (see Fig.4.7(a)). The ellipsoid is computed by solving

$$\frac{x_a^2}{\lambda_a^2} + \frac{x_b^2}{\lambda_b^2} + \frac{x_c^2}{\lambda_c^2} = 1. \tag{4.13}$$

x_i are Cartesian coordinates of a spherical unit vector.

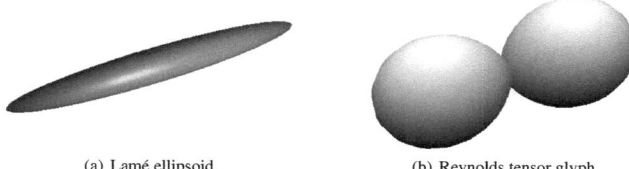

(a) Lamé ellipsoid   (b) Reynolds tensor glyph

Figure 4.7.: *Comparison: Lamé ellipsoid vs. Reynolds tensor glyph*

Another possibility to visualize diffusion tensor information is the *Reynolds tensor glyph* [43, 66]. The Reynolds tensor glyph will also orient itself according to the principal diffusion directions. The shape results from the inner product of the diffusion tensor with spherical unit vectors as described in (4.14).

$$\begin{aligned} r &= \mathbf{n}^T \mathbf{D} \mathbf{n} = \mathbf{D}_{\alpha\beta} \mathbf{n}_\alpha \mathbf{n}_\beta \\ &= \mathbf{D}_{xx}\mathbf{n}_x^2 + 2\mathbf{D}_{xy}\mathbf{n}_x\mathbf{n}_y + 2\mathbf{D}_{xz}\mathbf{n}_x\mathbf{n}_z + \mathbf{D}_{yy}\mathbf{n}_y^2 + 2\mathbf{D}_{yz}\mathbf{n}_y\mathbf{n}_z + \mathbf{D}_{zz}\mathbf{n}_z^2, \end{aligned} \tag{4.14}$$

with r the radius of the glyph, $\mathbf{D}_{\alpha\beta}$ a tensor element, and $\mathbf{n}_\alpha$ the Cartesian coordinates of a spherical unit vector [43]. The projections corresponding to these vectors are ideally distributed equally over the whole sphere so as not to bias the directionality of the glyph. This glyph is a peanut shape (see Fig.4.7(b)) which is similar to the ADC glyph (Fig.4.2; see also appendix D for a description of this similarity). By applying this method, each point on the surface of the glyph represents the diffusion strength in this direction according to (4.2). The diffusivity is accordingly directly proportional to the size of the glyph.

Both glyphs are similarly orientated along the axis of the eigenvector corresponding to the largest eigenvalue. The radii in both glyphs for the principal diffusion directions given by the eigenvectors are equal to the corresponding eigenvalues of the diffusion tensor.

The handling of large tensor data sets is facilitated by apt coloring of the tensor glyphs. The orientation of the glyph can be color coded by associating the principal eigenvector with RGB values (see for example Fig.4.8). This enables the viewer to directly grasp the orientation of the individual tensor in a larger tensor field. The tensor field visualization is often superimposed on an anatomic image of the measured subject to help the user put the information into context. In addition, the anisotropy can be coded in the intensity values of the diffusion glyph visualization rendering highly anisotropic regions lighter than more isotropic ones. This is illustrated in Fig.4.8, where the anisotropy is high, the ellipsoids are cigar shaped. Some examples are in the red/yellow bows of the corpus callosum in the center and top of the image. The more isotropic the diffusion inside a voxel is, the more spherical the corresponding ellipsoid will be. This is illustrated for example in the (mainly) dark liquor filled ventricles running top-down in the center of the figure, in which the diffusion is not restricted by any anatomical structures. The mean diffusivity in this region is still high but equally strong in all directions. This causes the ellipsoids to overlap, so no clear boundary can be detected here.

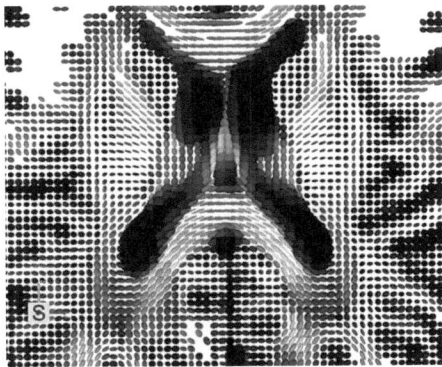

Figure 4.8.: *An example for the tensor visualization of the diffusion with lamé ellipsoids. For better orientation in the data set the intensity of the ellipsoid glyphs is coded according to the corresponding FA values and colored according to the orientation of their main axis.*

4.3. Recent Developments In Diffusion Evaluation

To overcome the limits of the standard second order diffusion tensor model, more advanced methods for the evaluation of HARDI data sets with a large number of diffusion encoding directions were proposed. These methods can be separated into two groups, advanced representation models, for example spherical harmonic decomposition (section 4.3.1) or multi-tensor representations (section 4.3.2), and advanced diffusion models, such as for example higher order diffusion tensors (section 4.3.3) or multi-compartment

4. Interpreting The Measured Diffusion

diffusion models (see for example [4]) (which will not be further discussed here). In the following, some of these more advanced methods are introduced in more detail.

4.3.1. Characterizing Diffusion With Spherical Harmonic Decomposition

A spherical harmonic decomposition (SHD) was proposed to characterize diffusion in HARDI data sets [32]. This approach is motivated by the inherent spherical symmetry in the HARDI measurements. This symmetry does not distinguish between diffusion in positive or negative gradient direction, both return the same signal ($S_\mathbf{g} = S_{-\mathbf{g}}$).

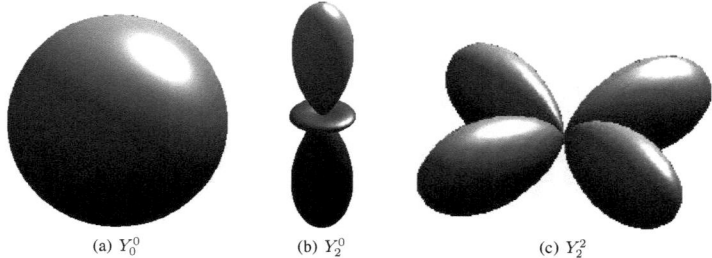

(a) Y_0^0 (b) Y_2^0 (c) Y_2^2

Figure 4.9.: *Examples for spherical harmonics*

The diffusion measurements can be expressed as a sum of rotations in three dimensional space relative to an unknown principal axis system of the diffusion. When the corresponding rotation matrices are transformed into a spherical space ($\mathbf{e} = r, \theta, \phi$, with r, the radius, θ the polar angle, between a vector and the positive Z-axis, and ϕ the azimuthal angle, relative to the positive X-axis), they are spherical harmonics [32]. Some examples for spherical harmonics are given in Fig.4.9. In spherical coordinates (θ, ϕ) the measured diffusion tensor can be expanded in a Laplace series of spherical harmonics Y_L^M:

$$\mathbf{D}(\theta, \phi) = \sum_{L=0}^{\infty} \sum_{M=-L}^{L} a_{LM} Y_L^M(\theta, \phi) \quad (4.15)$$

where $\mathbf{D}(\theta, \phi)$ gives the diffusion in direction (θ, ϕ). M is the order and L the degree of the spherical harmonic (Frank refers to L as the order of the spherical harmonic [32]). The coefficient a_{LM} is given by

$$a_{LM} = \int_0^{2\pi} \int_0^{\pi} \mathbf{D}(\theta, \phi) Y_L^M(\theta, \phi) sin(\theta) d\theta d\phi. \quad (4.16)$$

The odd degree of the spherical harmonics in the decomposition represent asymmetric parts in the signal which are assumed to be non-physical and, therefore, are considered artifacts. Artifacts that may result for example from motion of the subject, eddy currents

4.3. Recent Developments In Diffusion Evaluation

or measurement noise can be reduced by considering only the coefficients of even degree in the evaluation of diffusion. This should improve the evaluation even though the artifacts will partially remain in the reconstruction since they affect all degrees of the results from the SDH.

SHD is able to classify the diffusion in voxels in a HARDI data into three major categories: isotropic, single-fiber and multiple-fiber components (as illustrated in Fig.4.10) according to the the spherical harmonics Y_L^M used to describe the tensor.

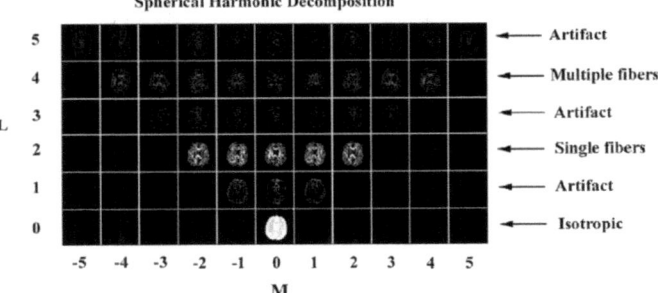

Figure 4.10.: *The different orders of SHD are illustrated here. L and M corresponds to the spherical harmonic basis Y_M^L. The degree of the decomposition L indicates the underlying voxel fiber structure as indicated on the right. Odd degrees of the decomposition are assumed contain only artifacts. This graphic is taken from [32].*

The first two categories (isotropic and single-fiber) can be adequately described by the regular second order diffusion tensor. The third category contains heterodirectional voxels, in this case the fiber orientation cannot be determined without specific assumptions on the fiber structure. Frank suggests the use of previous knowledge on the local anatomy to determine the fiber constellation with the highest probability [32]. If the number of fiber populations with different orientation in a heterodirectional voxel is given or chosen, their constellation can be reconstructed with the multi-tensor fit approaches similar to the one discussed in the next section.

4.3.2. Multi-Tensor Approach

This technique uses a given number of second order diffusion tensors to represent the measured diffusion. It is based on the definition of the measured signal in case of multiple fiber populations inside a single voxel (see (4.8)):

$$S_\mathbf{g} = S_0 * \sum \alpha_i F_i(\mathbf{g}) \qquad (4.17)$$
$$= S_0 * \sum \alpha_i exp(-b\mathbf{g}^T \mathbf{D}^i \mathbf{g}). \qquad (4.18)$$

4. Interpreting The Measured Diffusion

Here, α_i is the volume fraction corresponding to fiber population i. This fiber bundle produces the signal $F_i(\mathbf{g})$ for the gradient direction $\mathbf{g}$. The diffusion that corresponds to this fiber bundle can be adequately described with the corresponding second order tensor $\mathbf{D}^i$. As before, b stands for the diffusion weighting factor, $S_\mathbf{g}$ is the DWI signal and S_0 is the image without diffusion weighting. The difference between the signal estimated for a given tensors set and the measured signal is minimized to determine the set of tensors and volume fractions that describes the measured signal best. In [91], a given number of equally anisotropic cigar shaped tensors is used in the optimization. The individual tensors are assumed to be equal in shape to reduce the number of free parameters for the optimization, so the problem is solvable. A detailed description of the gradient descend used in this optimization is given in the appendix of [91]. Another approach [54] assumes that each voxel has some isotropic component that accounts for PVE in the measurement and two anisotropic components. Adding an isotropic tensor allows the two anisotropic tensors used in this approach to be relatively sharp cigars without diminishing the quality of the estimated multi-tensor signal fit to the measured signal. The measured signal is 'sharpened' by the subtraction of the isotropic components. This facilitates the fitting of highly anisotropic tensors to the remaining sharp signal. To ensure numerical stability of the optimization process the number of anisotropic tensors used in [54] was limited to two.

4.3.3. Generalized Diffusion Tensor Imaging

Another approach is describing the diffusion process with a generalized diffusion equation that uses higher order tensors (HOT) in the characterization of the diffusion process [74, 73, 57]. Non-Gaussian diffusion in heterodirectional voxels can be described with these HOTs. The HOT description of the diffusion in heterodirectional voxels can be more clearly represent multiple prominent diffusion directions than common DTI or even most HARDI reconstruction techniques [57]. HOT is still mainly used for probability density function (PDF) plots representing the individual voxels' diffusion profile. The HOT formalisms can be divided into two basic categories according to their data analysis techniques. The single HOT model [73] relies on the analysis of the ADC (similar to SHD) whereas the HOT hierarchy [57] is consistent with QSI.

4.3.3.1. The Single Higher Order Tensor Model

The single HOT model proposed by Özarslan and Mareci [73] assumes that the diffusion is restricted to the real-valued magnitude signal information. For the computation of this HOT model the Stejskal-Tanner relation is generalized to higher order tensors enabling straight forward calculation of all the coefficients with a least-squares fitting routine. A single HOT is fitted to the HARDI data:

$$S_\mathbf{g} = S_0 exp(-b\mathbf{g}_\alpha \mathbf{g}_\beta ... \mathbf{D}_{\alpha\beta...}). \qquad (4.19)$$

This equation is a direct extension of (4.3). The estimation matrix is accordingly generalized to contain the elements $\mathbf{B}_{\alpha\beta...} = -b\mathbf{g}_\alpha \mathbf{g}_\beta ...$ similar to the second order tensor

4.3. Recent Developments In Diffusion Evaluation

estimation matrix defined in (4.6). This tensor model is only defined for even tensor orders (odd orders are assumed to contain only artifact similar to the ones in the SHD). The tensor is symmetric similar to the second order tensor. This means all permutations of the indices are the same ($\mathbf{D}_{\alpha\beta\gamma\delta} = \mathbf{D}_{\alpha\beta\delta\gamma} = \ldots$). The symmetric HOT has $[(n+1)(n+2)]/2$ independent elements, with n the order of the tensor. The elements of lower order tensors of this model are related to the elements of the tensor of higher order and can therefore be easily computed from higher order tensor elements without refitting of the signal [73]. This facilitates a comparison of the results of different tensor orders. Some higher order anisotropy measures [74] were proposed to facilitate the interpretation of the data. The scalar measures can be used similar to the FA maps in the second order tensor evaluations.

Liu et al did show that models based on ADC analysis are mathematically self-inconsistent in presence of non-Gaussian diffusion [59]. ADC relies on the assumption that the MR-signal decays mono-exponentially as a function of a single b-value ($ADC_g = b^{-1} ln(S_g/S_0)$). In the presence of non-Gaussian diffusion a mono-exponential decay does not exist for every diffusion encoding gradient direction. The ADC in these cases is, therefore, not well defined. This is the reason for problems of ADC based reconstruction methods, for example the insufficient reconstruction of the underlying fiber orientations in heterodirectional voxels [59]. In spite of this, the model can still be used to determine heterogeneous regions and obtain at least some information on the fiber constellation successfully [26].

4.3.3.2. The Higher Order Tensor Hierarchy

The HOT hierarchy model developed by Liu et al is based on $\mathbf{q}$-space imaging [58, 57, 59]. The signal S is interpreted, similarly to the introduction in 3.4, as

$$S = S_0 \int \overline{P_s}(\mathbf{R}, \Delta) \, exp\left(-i\mathbf{qR}\right) d\mathbf{R}. \tag{4.20}$$

i is the imaginary unit ($i^2 = -1$), $\mathbf{q} = \gamma\delta\mathbf{G}$ and $\mathbf{R} = \mathbf{r}' - \mathbf{r}$ as defined in 3.4. If the random variable $\mathbf{R}$ is distributed asymmetrically the signal S is complex valued according to (4.20) [59].

S/S_0 is the characteristic function of the random variable $\mathbf{R}$ with the probability density function $\overline{P_s}(\mathbf{R}, \Delta)$. The cumulants of the random variable $\mathbf{R}$ can be used to expand the characteristic function to:

$$\frac{S}{S_0} = exp\left(\frac{(-i)Q^1_{j_1} q_{j_1}}{1!} + \frac{(-i)^2 Q^2_{j_1 j_2} q_{j_1} q_{j_2}}{2!} + \cdots + \frac{(-i)^n Q^n_{j_1 j_2 \ldots j_n} q_{j_1} q_{j_2} \cdots q_{j_n}}{n!}\right) \tag{4.21}$$

The coefficients $Q^n_{j_1 j_2 \ldots j_n}$ are the nth order cumulants of $\mathbf{R}$,

$$\mathbf{Q}^{(n)}_{j_1 j_2 \ldots j_n} \approx n! \mathbf{D}^{(n)}_{j_1 j_2 \ldots j_n} \Delta. \tag{4.22}$$

Δ is the separation time of the two diffusion gradients and δ the duration of the individual

4. Interpreting The Measured Diffusion

gradients. Then (4.21) can be rewritten as:

$$S = S_0 exp(\sum_{n=2}^{\infty} i^n \mathbf{g}_{j_1} \mathbf{g}_{j_2} ... \mathbf{g}_{j_n} \mathbf{D}^{(n)}_{j_1 j_2 ... j_n} b^{(n)}). \quad (4.23)$$

D^n is the tensor of order n and b^n is the diffusion weighting factor that corresponds to the tensor order n. $\mathbf{g}$ is the diffusion encoding gradient direction with components j_n ($j \in x, y, z$). The diffusion weighting factors in (4.23) are an extension of (3.13) for an arbitrary tensor order n.

$$b^n = \gamma^n G^n \delta^n (\Delta - \frac{n-1}{n+1}\delta), \quad (4.24)$$

They do depend on the measurement parameters δ, Δ, γ and G used in the data acquisition (as defined in section 3.3) but only b^2 is equal to the diffusion weighting factor used as parameter for the MR-scanner.

The equation system that needs to be solved to estimate the diffusion tensors is similar to (4.5). The rows of the estimation matrix $\mathbf{B}$ have to be adjusted to support the larger number of b-factors. The row corresponding to direction i is given by:

$$d^i = \begin{bmatrix} b^2 g^i_{xx} b^2 g^i_{yy} \cdots j b^3 g^i_{xxx} \cdots - b^4 g^i_{xxxx} \cdots \end{bmatrix}. \quad (4.25)$$

This tensor model is evaluated on the complete complex-valued measured signal. All other advanced evaluation methods work on the magnitude signals only. The model does not make any assumptions on the diffusion process [57]. Consequently, all higher order tensors, odd and even ordered, are important to the reconstruction.

This tensor model is able to reconstruct the fiber orientation accurately. An advantage in this model is the handling of asymmetric fiber constellation, such as Y-shaped fiber branching. The asymmetric diffusion properties needed to resolve this geometry are revealed in the signal phase. If the phase is ignored, as it is done in other models, the asymmetry information is lost. In the HOT hierarchy this information is stored in tensors of odd order. The asymmetry of the resulting PDF for the reconstruction seems to be a clear violation of the principle of microscopic detailed balance, this principle needs to be broken down in voxel imaging for an accurate representation of the non-Gaussian diffusion process [59]. The non-Gaussianity of the measured diffusion originates from the limited spatial imaging resolution that results in PVE in heterogeneous voxels and the fact that the measured diffusion is not free but hindered.

The asymmetric parts of the signal are coded in the imaginary part of the complex signal which will be zero if the signal is completely symmetric. Symmetric structures such as crossing fibers are coded in the real part of the signal. The incorporation of the odd order tensors will cause a shift in the diffusion profile. For a Y-shaped fiber, for example, the two lower corners of the square glyph in Fig.4.11(b) are forced inwards by the odd order tensor to form the Y. A comparison of glyphs corresponding to different parts of the hierarchy is given in Fig.4.11. All glyphs in Fig.4.11 correspond to the same Y-shaped anatomy. Fig.4.11(a) shows the corresponding disc shaped second order glyph that allows only one dominating diffusion direction. This direction does not correspond to any arm of the Y-shape. In Fig.4.11(b) only even order tensors from the hierarchy

4.3. Recent Developments In Diffusion Evaluation

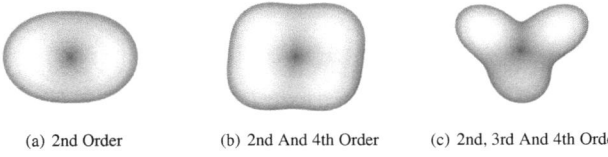

(a) 2nd Order (b) 2nd And 4th Order (c) 2nd, 3rd And 4th Order

Figure 4.11.: *The influence of the odd order tensor on the PDF is illustrated.*

are used to reconstruct the anatomy, resulting in a symmetric square shape similar to a glyph corresponding to fiber crossing. The corners of this glyph correspond to the orientations of the upper two arms of the Y-shape. The even order tensor information is always symmetric therefore the asymmetric Y-shape cannot be reconstructed. The complete reconstruction with even and odd order tensors is shown in Fig.4.11(c). The two lower corners are forced inwards to form the Y-shape.

The reconstruction of Y-shaped fibers is only relevant if the Y clearly dominates the voxel. This is usually not the case in the voxel size that can be acquired in DTI today. The three arms of the Y will usually dominate over the small region where the fiber is actually branching. Even though the voxel volume in images acquired today are probably too large to render the case of Y-shaped fibers important, the ability to handle asymmetric diffusion is a theoretical advantage of this tensor model over the previously presented single HOT model.

The HOT hierarchy of maximal tensor order four has 31 independent tensor elements. 31 is, therefore, the minimal required number of encoding directions. To improve the stability of the tensor estimation, several diffusion weighted measurements with different weighting factors were suggested [57].

Results From My HOT Hierarchy Evaluations It is a property of this hierarchical model that all real part information is contained in the even order tensors and all information from the imaginary part of the signal in the odd order tensors [58]. I was therefore able to estimate the tensors for this model from two smaller equation systems, one for each part of the signal (real and imaginary). A row of the even order estimation matrix is for example given by:

$$d^i = \begin{bmatrix} b^2 g^i_{xx} b^2 g^i_{yy} \cdots - b^4 g^i_{xxxx} \cdots \end{bmatrix}. \quad (4.26)$$

This will reduce the maximal required rank in the estimation matrix. The estimation matrix needs to have a rank equal the maximal number of independent tensor elements that are to be estimated by one of the equation systems (even or odd order).

$$rank = max(\sum_{n=2j}^{N} \frac{(n+1)(n+2)}{2}, \sum_{n=2j+1}^{N} \frac{(n+1)(n+2)}{2}), j = 1...N/2. \quad (4.27)$$

$rank$ gives the required rank for the estimation matrix, n is the tensor order and N is the maximal tensor order used in this evaluation. The minimal number of required gradient encoding directions is reduced with the rank of the estimation matrix. For a maximal tensor order of four the required number of directions is reduced from 31 (6 for the second order, 10 for the third and 15 for the fourth) to 21 (6 plus 15). The imaginary part of 21 acquired directions is more than enough for the estimation of 10 independent elements of the third order tensor. This is a considerable improvement in the required number of measurements and therefore also reduces the time needed for the data acquisition.

Liu showed in [57] that he could reconstruct the HOT hierarchy with a single b-factor greater zero. However, a single b-factor is only sufficient if a large number of encoding directions ($N_e \geq 200$) is used. In my investigations I found that for a low number of encoding directions ($N_e < 100$) the equation system for the tensor estimation with a single b-factor does not have full rank. If the rank of the estimation matrix is not full, the tensors cannot be estimated, because no unique solution exists. When at least two b-factors larger zero are used, the rank of the estimation matrix is always full. The use of at least two b-factors larger zero is advantageous because two acquisitions of a low number of encoding directions with different b-factors are usually faster than one acquisition with a considerably larger number of encoding directions. The optimal choice of the two b-factors still needs to be determined.

4.3.3.3. Visualization Of The Higher Order Tensors

For the visualization of the HOT hierarchy diffusion profile an established technique, visualizing the probability density function (PDF) P corresponding to the diffusion model can be used. First, a unit sphere around the origin (0,0,0) is generated. Each point on the sphere represents a direction **r** in 3D space. Then the PDF corresponding to the tensor representation of the DTI signals, is evaluated for each of these directions. The result is the radius rad of the glyph in the direction **r**.

$$rad(\mathbf{r}) = P(\mathbf{r}) \tag{4.28}$$

This glyph representation has great similarities with the Reynolds glyph for second order tensors (4.14).

The PDF of the single HOT approach is given by the estimated tensor. The surface is therefore computed with

$$P(\mathbf{r}) = \mathbf{D}(\mathbf{r}) = \sum_{\alpha=1}^{3} \sum_{\beta=1}^{3} ... \mathbf{D}_{\alpha\beta...} \mathbf{r}_\alpha \mathbf{r}_\beta .... \tag{4.29}$$

This equation is a straight forward generalization of the Reynolds glyph (4.14).

The PDF for the HOT hierarchy can be described by a Gram-Chalier series [64] which is a common method for the definition of a PDF of a random variable with its higher order statistics. The PDF of **r** for the HOT hierarchy is therefore defined as

$$P(\mathbf{r}) = N(0, \mathbf{Q}_{kl}^{(2)})(1 + \frac{\mathbf{Q}_{klm}^{(3)} \mathbf{H}^{klm}(\mathbf{r})}{3!} + \frac{\mathbf{Q}_{klmn}^{(4)} \mathbf{H}^{klmn}(\mathbf{r})}{4!} + ...) \tag{4.30}$$

4.3. Recent Developments In Diffusion Evaluation

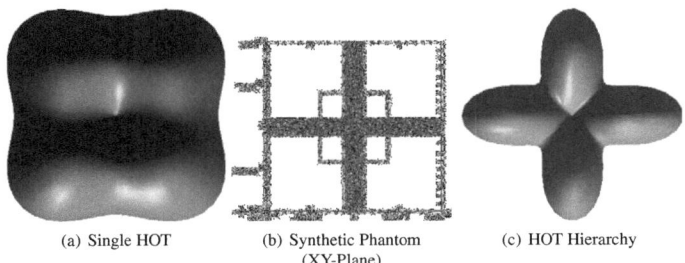

(a) Single HOT (b) Synthetic Phantom (XY-Plane) (c) HOT Hierarchy

Figure 4.12.: *An example for the two kinds of HOT glyph for a pair of orthogonally crossing fibers. The HOTs were estimated from simulated data sets without noise and an force-minimizing encoding scheme [50] with 81 directions. (b) shows a cross-sectional cut through the synthetic phantom evaluated here (image adopted from [57]). The position of the evaluated voxel is indicated by the stippled line.*

$N(0, \mathbf{Q}_{kl}^{(2)})$ describes the normal density distribution with covariance matrix, $\mathbf{Q}_{kl}^{(2)}$, and zero mean. The notation $\mathbf{Q}_{klm}\mathbf{H}^{klm}(\mathbf{r})$ is used as short form of the Einstein summation convention,

$$\mathbf{Q}_{klm}\mathbf{H}^{klm}(\mathbf{r}) = \sum_{k=1}^{3}\sum_{l=1}^{3}\sum_{m=1}^{3} \mathbf{Q}_{klm}\mathbf{H}^{klm}(\mathbf{r}). \tag{4.31}$$

$\mathbf{H}^{i_1 i_2 \ldots i_n}(\mathbf{r})$ is the n-th order Hermite tensor [64]. The Hermite tensors up to order four are given using the Einstein summation rule described in (4.31):

$$\begin{aligned}
H^k &= N(0, \mathbf{Q}_{kl}^{(2)})^{-1} \\
H^{kl} &= H^k H^l - N(0, \mathbf{Q}_{kl}^{(2)})^{-1} \\
H^{klm} &= H^k H^l H^m - H^k N(0, \mathbf{Q}_{lm}^{(2)})^{-1} \\
H^{klmn} &= H^k H^l H^m H^n - H^k H^l N(0, \mathbf{Q}_{mn}^{(2)})^{-1} + N(0, \mathbf{Q}_{kl}^{(2)})^{-1} N(0, \mathbf{Q}_{mn}^{(2)})^{-1}.
\end{aligned} \tag{4.32}$$

A comparison of the diffusion glyphs for both HOT models illustrates the superiority of the reconstruction of the diffusion orientation in the HOT hierarchy. Fig.4.12 compares the two HOT models for a voxel containing two orthogonally crossing fibers. This fiber constellation is symmetric and should, therefore, be reconstructible for the single HOT model as well as for the HOT hierarchy. The glyph corresponding to the single HOT (Fig.4.12(a)) does not much resemble the input geometry (Fig.4.12(b)). The main axes of the PDF glyph do not correspond to the fibers in Fig.4.12(c). The HOT hierarchy PDF glyph on the other side reconstructs the fibers accurately. Another example is given in Fig.4.13. This asymmetric Y-shape is not resolvable for the single HOT model. It is therefore not surprising that Fig.4.13(a) and Fig.4.13(b) have not much in common. The HOT hierarchy glyph is for this case also able to reconstruct the axes of the fibers accurately.

4. Interpreting The Measured Diffusion

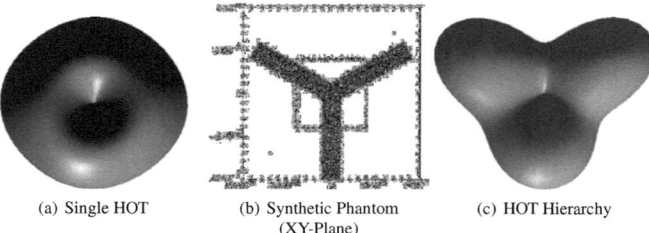

(a) Single HOT   (b) Synthetic Phantom (XY-Plane)   (c) HOT Hierarchy

Figure 4.13.: *A comparison of the diffusion glyphs of the two presented HOT models for a splitting fiber. The HOTs were estimated from simulated data sets without noise and an force-minimizing encoding scheme [50] with 21 directions. (b) shows a cross-sectional cut through the synthetic phantom used to simulate the data evaluated here (image adopted from [57]). The position of the evaluated voxel is indicated by a stippled square.*

Fig.4.14 compares the different HOT models for different numbers of encoding directions. The directions corresponding to extrema in the PDF surface are color coded. The coordinates of the extrema are translated into RGB values. This pronounces the deviation of the reconstructed diffusion directions from the one in the input signal in Fig.4.14(a). It can be seen that the reconstructed diffusion directions for the single HOT model Fig.4.14(b) do not correspond well to the input diffusion directions (Fig.4.14(a)). Even with an increase in measured directions, which should result in an increased reconstruction quality, there is no improvement in the reconstruction of the orientations. The directions reconstructed by the HOT hierarchy Fig.4.14(c) fit the input directions much better and some increase in quality is observable with an increase in encoding directions.

4.3. Recent Developments In Diffusion Evaluation

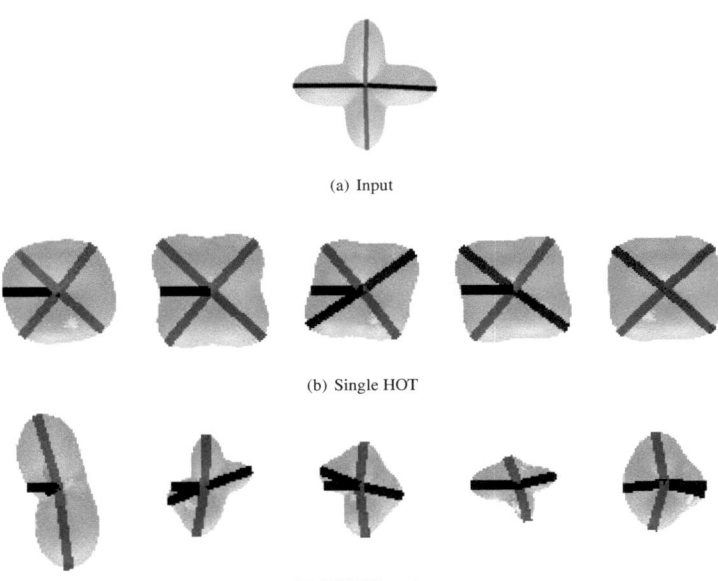

(a) Input

(b) Single HOT

(c) HOT Hierarchy

Figure 4.14.: *A comparison of the diffusion glyphs. The lines give the extrema of the corresponding reconstructed PDF, which correspond to dominating diffusion directions. In (a) the input glyph is given. Below the evaluation with the single HOT (b) and the HOT hierarchy (c) are given with an increasing number of encoding directions from left to right ($N_e = 21, 30, 46, 81, 126$). The evaluations were performed on simulated data sets with SNR 20 and an force-minimizing encoding scheme [50].*

5. Gradient Encoding Schemes

For DTI the number of diffusion weighting gradient directions has to be at least equal to the number of free parameters in the chosen tensor model. In the following, 'encoding direction' or 'gradient directions' is used as short form of 'diffusion weighting gradient direction'.

For the tensor estimation a linear equation system of the form

$$\mathbf{D} = \mathbf{B}^{-1}\mathbf{Y} \qquad (5.1)$$

has to be solved (see section 4.2 for more details). The vector $\mathbf{D}$ contains the independent tensor elements to be estimated. The dimension of $\mathbf{D}$ depends on the tensor model that is used. $\mathbf{B}$ is the estimation matrix describing the diffusion weighting. It contains the information on the encoding directions used in a gradient encoding scheme (GES). For details on the construction of the estimation matrix see chapter 4. $\mathbf{Y}$ contains the measured signal ($ln(S_g/S_0)$). The estimation matrix $\mathbf{B}$ needs to have full rank to guarantee the existence of an unique solution for (5.1) [88]. It was proposed that to ensure high quality estimation results, the distribution of the encoding directions over the sphere should well approximate equidistribution [47, 49, 76, 84]. It is argued that a set of directions that is well distributed over the unit sphere will optimize the tensor estimation results for an arbitrary tensor orientation.

For the investigation of chosen known fiber bundles, or parts thereof, one can use prior knowledge on the anatomy to optimize the quality of the estimated tensor for the chosen fiber orientation. A strategy to do so was proposed by Peng and Arfanakis [80]. This method performs better for the chosen fiber orientation but the quality decreases significantly for fibers that are not aligned with the chosen orientation. The method is therefore only suitable for the investigation of certain preselected fiber bundles or pieces thereof which are similarly oriented. It cannot be used for whole brain investigations and is especially unsuitable for the investigation of tracts for which the fiber orientation is not known prior to the measurement.

The goal of my work is the identification of well performing GES for arbitrary fiber orientations. Therefore, I concentrate on the optimization of the equidistribution of the gradient directions over the whole sphere to allow good tensor estimation for any tensor orientation.

The ideal diffusion encoding scheme would sample the unit sphere at an infinitesimally large number of points to guarantee that all directions are equally well represented [10]. This ideal cannot be achieved in actual discrete measurements, this is why each encoding scheme is only an approximation of the ideal sphere-sampling. Today, it is also not possible to generate a true equidistribution for an arbitrary number of points on a sphere. This is as far as I know still one of the unsolved problems in mathematics [30].

There are many ways to generate a gradient encoding scheme with a sufficiently high number of directions. In the following, some of the encoding schemes known from literature will be presented.

5.1. Polyhedral Encoding Schemes

A natural way to achieve a regular distribution over the unit sphere is to resort to geometry, especially to regular polyhedra. The family of regular polyhedra includes, for example, the tetrahedron, the cube, the octahedron and the icosahedron. The encoding schemes based on these geometric structures choose their encoding directions to be either the vertices of a polyhedron or the ones of a related refinement, which generate more regular distributed points on the sphere. The so constructed gradient encoding schemes can be combined to create new encoding schemes with even more directions (see for example in [10, 52]).

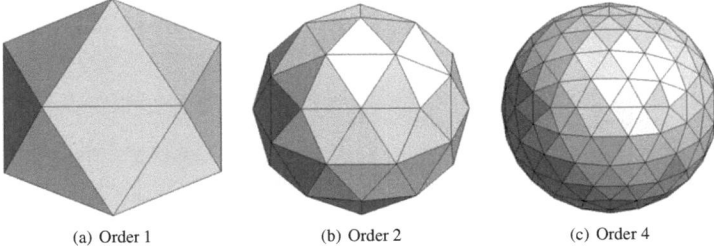

(a) Order 1 (b) Order 2 (c) Order 4

Figure 5.1.: *This figure shows some examples for the triangulation of the regular icosahedron as means for mesh refinement.*

Here, I concentrate on geometric constructions based on the regular icosahedron (see Fig.5.1(a)) consisting of twelve vertices and twenty triangular faces. Each vertex of a regular symmetrical polyhedron has a corresponding vertex on the opposite hemisphere. These two points can be connected by a straight line through the approximated sphere's origin. Under the assumption that $S_\mathbf{g} = S_{-\mathbf{g}}$ only the vertices on one hemisphere are used in the GES. The vertices of the regular icosahedron, therefore, correspond to six non-collinear gradient directions. This GES with six directions is often used for the estimation of the standard second order diffusion tensor. It has been shown that no gradient encoding scheme with the minimal required six diffusion gradient directions is superior to the regular icosahedron for the computation of the second order diffusion tensor [10, 42, 70].

When the icosahedral mesh is refined by triangulation (see Fig.5.1 and 5.2(b)), the number of encoding directions is $N_e = 5n^2 + 1$, with n the order of the triangulation

5. Gradient Encoding Schemes

($n = 1, 2, 3, ...$). n^2 is the number of new faces after triangulation for each old face [42]. The sampling of the sphere is improved with increased triangulation order.

Other methods of refinement that are usually also referred to as icosahedral GES are presented in the following. Their relation to the regular icosahedron is illustrated in Fig.5.2. One refinement method exploits the dual relationship between the regular icosahedron and the dodecahedron whose vertices correspond to the centroids of the regular icosaeder's faces (see Fig.5.2(c)). The transformation of the regular icosahedron to a regular dodecahedron increases the number of encoding directions from six to ten.

By bisecting the edges of icosahedral polygons new regular shapes are created, which can be used to find encoding schemes with more directions. An example with 15 directions results from the edge bisection of the basic regular icosahedron (see Fig.5.2(d)). The geometry of the spherical fullerene, C_{60}, also known as bucky (soccer) ball, is the result of vertex truncation, skipping certain vertices of a refined icosahedral mesh. The corresponding point distribution was shown to be a true equidistribution on the sphere [23]. An example for a combination of direction sets to generate GES with even more directions is a scheme with 16 directions that results from the combination of the icosahedral and dodecahedral vertices.

In the illustrations in Fig.5.2 it can be seen that not all refined meshes result in equally well distributed sets of vertices. For example, the vertices resulting from edge bisection (Fig.5.2(d)) are not optimally spread, i.e. the distance between the vertices is not maximal. The vertices of the icosahedron which was used as base for this refinement lie in a 'hole' of the new mesh, the surrounding new vertices have each four neighbors but do not include the old vertices. The dodecahedron (Fig.5.2(c)) seems to have similar 'holes', but vertices in this refinement are overall well spread. This phenomenon needs to be taken into account. The estimation based on an encoding scheme resulting from bisection might be biased because of the inferior spread of directions even though it is related to the generally well spread family of icosahedral encoding schemes.

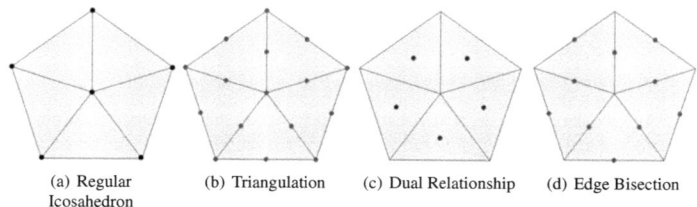

(a) Regular Icosahedron (b) Triangulation (c) Dual Relationship (d) Edge Bisection

Figure 5.2.: *Examples for the refinement of the icosahedral mesh. The dots give the position of the vertices of the refinement.*

The icosahedral schemes in general are straight forward and easy to compute but they also have a major disadvantage. They are restricted in N_e. They cannot produce an arbitrary number of encoding directions. This is a disadvantage when the encoding scheme is supposed to minimize the number of encoding directions and thereby measurements.

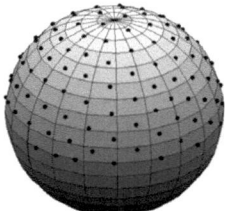

Figure 5.3.: *The points show the 126 encoding directions over the sphere that correspond to half the vertices of a refined icosahedron.*

The minimal number of encoding directions does not necessarily coincide with the N_e of an icosahedral scheme. Also the quality of the approximation of an equidistribution on the sphere with the icosahedral refinements is limited [23, 85]. This can be geometrically explained for the triangulation with the observation that the spherical triangles, resulting from the refinement, do not all cover equal areas [85]. This observation can be transferred to the other refinements since they are all related to the icosahedral triangulation. The vertices of the basic icosahedron, the basic dodecahedron and the *bucky ball* (Icosa30; a certain truncated triangulation of the basic icosahedron) are equidistributed over the sphere.

The GES whose directions are related to the regular icosahedron are referred to as Icosa further on. An example GES with 126 directions is given in Fig.5.3.

5.2. Analytical Schemes

One drawback for the geometrical encoding schemes is that they are only able to generate an arbitrary fixed number of encoding directions. To overcome this limitation and allow a reduction of the encoding direction overhead analytical methods for the distribution of an arbitrary number of directions were proposed.

Wong and Roos proposed to compute the components of the gradient vectors as follows [94]:

$$
\begin{aligned}
g_z(d) &= \frac{1}{N_e} 2d - N_e - 1 \\
g_x(d) &= \cos\left(\frac{\sqrt{N_e}\pi}{\sin(g_z(d))}\right) \sqrt{1 - g_z(d)^2} \\
g_y(d) &= \sqrt{1 - g_z(d)^2 - g_x(d)^2}.
\end{aligned}
\tag{5.2}
$$

Here, N_e is the total number of encoding directions and d is the index of the directions ($d = 1, 2, \ldots, N_e$). A large N_e is needed to get (reasonably) well distributed directions ($N_e \ll 6$). For smaller N_e the encoding directions are not well spread. This method is referred to as Ana1 in the results section. An example is given in Fig.5.4(a).

5. Gradient Encoding Schemes

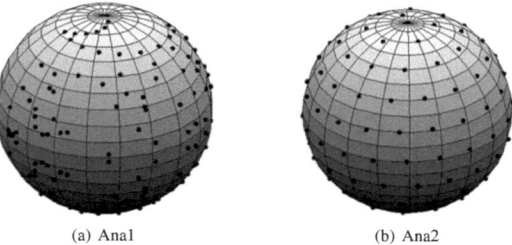

(a) Ana1   (b) Ana2

Figure 5.4.: *The points illustrate the distribution of the 126 encoding directions over the sphere as result of the analytical GES generation algorithms.*

The second analytical method presented here was proposed by Staff and Kuijlaars [85] and delivers a very good approximation of equidistribution for a chosen number of points on the unit sphere. It was inspired by the geometry of the perfectly distributed bucky ball.

$$\begin{aligned}
g_x(d) &= cos(\phi(d)) * sin(arccos(h(d))) \\
g_y(d) &= sin(\phi(d)) * sin(arccos(h(d))) \\
g_z(d) &= cos(arccos(h(d))) \\
h(d) &= -1 + 2 * \frac{d-1}{N_e - 1} \\
\phi(d) &= \begin{cases} 0 & \text{if } d \in \{1, N_e\} \\ mod(\phi(d-1) + \frac{3.6}{\sqrt{N_e * (1-h(d)^2)}}, 2\pi) & \text{else} \end{cases}
\end{aligned} \quad (5.3)$$

with N_e and d as defined before. This algorithm requires at least 10 directions to compute a satisfactory spread set of points. The distribution is best for N_e larger 30. The corresponding GES are named Ana2 later on. An example direction set is plotted in Fig.5.4(b).

5.3. Numerically Optimized Encoding Schemes

An alternative to the previously discussed GES creation methods is the distribution of N_e gradient directions on the unit sphere by numerical optimization according to a given criterion. In the following, some of the more prominent examples known from literature are presented.

5.3.1. Minimum Force Approach

The idea of the minimum force approach is to obtain a distribution of gradient directions which maximizes their separation by minimizing the corresponding forces between them

5.3. Numerically Optimized Encoding Schemes

[42, 49]. To do so, each gradient direction is associated with two projected points on the sphere (**g** and **-g**) as illustrated in Fig.5.5(a). An electrostatic force is assumed to exist between all thus defined points on the sphere. This force is proportional to the distance between the points, **g**. The total force for the whole GES is equal to the sum of the forces between the individual points. This translates to the following optimization criterion:

$$\epsilon = \sum_{i=1}^{2N_e} \sum_{j=1}^{2N_e} \frac{1}{\left\| \mathbf{g}^{(i)} - \mathbf{g}^{(j)} \right\|}. \tag{5.4}$$

The algorithm stops rearranging the directions when the sum of the force between the points ($\left\| \mathbf{g}^{(i)} - \mathbf{g}^{(j)} \right\|$)is minimal that means, the energy ϵ is maximized. The repulsion between the points is illustrated in Fig.5.5(a). The point corresponding to the inverse gradient direction is considered in the optimization process. Members of this encoding scheme family are labeled ForcePairs(N_e) in the following. An example for a ForcePairs126 GES is shown in Fig.5.6(a).

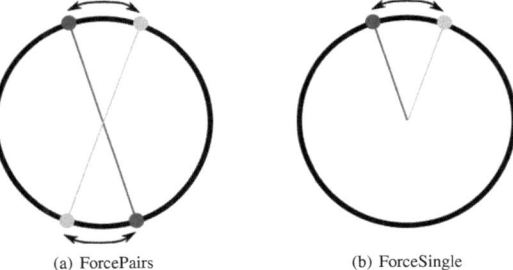

(a) ForcePairs (b) ForceSingle

Figure 5.5.: *An example for the repulsion between the points on the sphere.*

From mathematics a similar approach for the distribution of points on a sphere is known [30]. This approach does not use pairs connected through the origin in the optimization but optimizes the position of the individual points with the criterion in (5.4). The repulsion between the individual points is illustrated in Fig.5.5(b). The positions of the inverse gradient directions are not considered during the optimization of the directions. The so generated GES are called ForceSingle(N_e) further on. An example GES with 126 directions is plotted in Fig.5.6(b).

Both force-minimizing problems have multiple local minima. The optimization will return a distribution that is close to the global minimum [30] but cannot guarantee to return the actual global optimum. Approaches to find the global minimum have been introduced but all of them are unable to guarantee to return the global minimum for an arbitrary number of directions and are therefore disregarded in the following evaluations.

5. Gradient Encoding Schemes

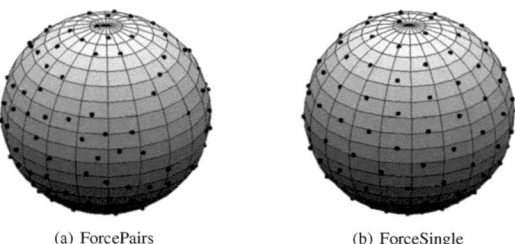

(a) ForcePairs (b) ForceSingle

Figure 5.6.: *An example for an force minimizing direction sets with 126 directions.*

5.3.2. Minimal Condition Number Algorithm

A different approach minimizes the condition number of the estimation matrix **B** to generate an encoding scheme [84]. The condition number is an indicator for the quality of an equation system which is solved numerically [88]. In the context of tensor estimation, it is an upper boundary for the error propagation from the right hand side of estimation equation system (5.1) to the tensor elements [84, 88].

The condition number can be easily computed from singular value decomposition of the estimation matrix $\mathbf{B} = \mathbf{U}\Sigma\mathbf{V}^T$ with **U** a column orthogonal matrix, Σ a diagonal matrix containing the singular values of **B** and **V** a square orthogonal matrix. The condition number κ is equal to the relation between the maximal and minimal singular value [88]:

$$\epsilon = \kappa(\mathbf{B}) = \frac{\max(\sigma)}{\min(\sigma)}. \tag{5.5}$$

The so optimized schemes are called "Cond(N_e)" in the following evaluations. An example GES with 126 directions is shown in Fig.5.7.

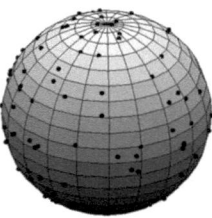

Figure 5.7.: *An example for a Cond GES with 126 directions.*

6. Determining The Quality Of Encoding Schemes

To determine which encoding scheme to use in a DTI or HARDI measurement, one needs to quantify its quality. The term 'quality' in this context means the ability to estimate a given tensor accurately from noisy data. In this chapter, several quality measures known from literature are presented. Some of these are evaluated for second or higher order tensor models later on. New quality measures are also investigated and compared with the established ones.

6.1. The Evaluated GES

For the condition number evaluation, the different gradient encoding schemes were evaluated for the single HOT model (section 4.3.3.1) up to order eight, which requires an estimation matrix with rank 45. The HOT hierarchy (section 4.3.3.2) was evaluated up to order six, requiring a rank of 49. These two maximal tensor orders were chosen because the number of independent tensor elements (rank) for both HOT models are close to each other for better comparison. The signal accuracy evaluation did investigate both HOT models for a maximal tensor order of four only.

The HOT hierarchy model could be successfully evaluated for only two different b-factors. The quality indices with two b-factors were of the same order of magnitude as the one for the ten b-factor estimation matrices used here. The actual condition number depends on the choice of b-factors. Since the optimal choice of b-factors is not yet defined, the b-factors used in this evaluation were computed according to (4.24) for $\delta = 30$ ms, $\Delta = 40$ ms and G increasing from 4 to 40 mT/m in ten equidistant steps (as suggested by Liu et al in [57]). This results in a maximal b-factor of ~ 3100 s/mm^2 corresponding to the second order tensor.

The condition number does not change for the single HOT model when multiple b-factors are used in the measurement. The condition number investigation of this tensor model was therefore performed for one b-factor only to allow faster computation. For the signal accuracy evaluation the same 10 b-factors used for the HOT hierarchy are used for all evaluated tensor models.

The Icosa GES cannot generate an arbitrary number of directions, because they are determined by the geometry of the regular icosahedron. The evaluation presented here is focused on a range of directions that can be measured on standard scanners in a rea-

6. Determining The Quality Of Encoding Schemes

sonable time span (less than an hour for one acquisition of a whole brain dataset with common voxel size Δx ($\Delta x > 1mm^3$)). Schemes with $N_e = 15, 16, 21, 30, 46, 81, 126$ were selected for the investigation. The minimal N_e was chosen to be 15 because this is the minimal required number of encoding directions for HOT evaluations (single HOT of order four). In section 6.4 and 6.6 $N_e = 6, 10$ were included in the second order tensor evaluation. All other GES were generated for these N_e to allow direct comparison.

No averaging was used since there is no reasonably small common multiple for the evaluated N_e. Jones showed that an increase in N_e outperforms an increase in the number of averages if the number of measurements is the same [47]. This question is therefore not further investigated here. Instead, I concentrated on the direct comparison of different GES creation methods for the same N_e.

The numerically optimized schemes vary with each optimization. I evaluated all numerically optimized schemes 100 times, each time initialized with a new set of random directions. The evaluation showed that the performance of each force-minimizing GES was close to the mean over all evaluations (which is in accordance with, for example, Staff and Kuijlaars [85]). Only one exemplary optimization for ForceSingle and Force-Pairs was used for the evaluation of GES quality because the individual optimizations are so very similar. The most variable GESs are COND schemes. The representative GES from this family was selected so that its behavior in the evaluation is close to the mean over 100 optimizations.

All evaluations were performed with MATLAB [1]) on standard PCs. The numerically optimized schemes were evaluated with the code available from the internet[2] or extensions thereof. The code for the calculation of the regular, even order, icosahedral triangulations was also taken from the internet [3]. The computations for all presented numerical optimization methods were terminated when the relative change between two successive optimization function values was less then 10^{-6}, or the maximum of 10^6 function evaluations or iterations was reached.

The Cond schemes were obtained by employing both, the standard second order estimation matrix and the higher order **B**-matrices, in the optimization function. The resulting schemes have full rank for all tensor models evaluated here regardless of the matrix used in the optimization as long as N_e is larger than the number of independent tensor elements. I found that the condition number and its standard deviation have approximately the same values for both approaches. The computation was considerably faster when the second order tensor estimation matrix was used in the optimization, which is why this matrix was employed for the generation of the Cond GES used here.

---

[1] Developed by the MathWorks, Inc.; MATLAB Version 7.1.0.246 (R14) Service Pack 3.
[2] Available on the homepage of Dr. Peter Batchelor, http://www.cs.ucl.ac.uk/staff/p.batchelor/dti-directions/dti-directions/.
[3] MATLAB schript sphere-tri.m from www.koders.com.

6.2. Known Indices

This chapter starts with the presentation of quality measures for the second order diffusion tensor estimation known from literature. Different ways to quantify the quality of an encoding scheme were proposed, some are based on the quantification of the error propagation in the estimation process [42, 76, 84] and others on the quality of the spread of the GES directions [52, 70].

6.2.1. Total Variance

An index ν to quantify the stability of the tensor estimation was proposed by Papadakis et al [76]. ν is a scalar measure which is proportional to the total variance of the diffusion tensor in an isotropic medium if all DWI were measured with the same b-factors. To generate ν, the covariance matrix $\mathbf{F}$ of the inverse estimation matrix $\mathbf{B}^{-1}$ ($\mathbf{F} = \mathbf{B}^{-1}\mathbf{B}^{-T}$) needs to be computed, first. $\mathbf{F}$ describes the propagation of uncorrelated errors in the estimation from the $\overline{ADC}$ vector $\mathbf{Y}$ (see (4.5)) to the elements of the diffusion tensor $\mathbf{D}$. A property of covariance matrices is that their diagonal elements give the variance of the individual random variables. Here the investigated random variables are the rows $\mathbf{B}^{-1}$ which contain information on the gradient encoding directions. The total variance of the tensor $\mathbf{D}$ is the sum the variance of its elements, that is the sum of the diagonal elements of $\mathbf{F}$. The index ν is then defined for the second order tensor as follows:

$$\nu = tr(\mathbf{F}) + \mathbf{F}_{44} + \mathbf{F}_{55} + \mathbf{F}_{66}. \tag{6.1}$$

Note that $\mathbf{F}$ for the second order tensor model is a 6x6 matrix and the diagonal elements give the variance of the 6 tensor elements of the 3x3 diffusion tensor. Because the off-diagonal elements appear twice in the second order diffusion tensor, their corresponding error terms ($\mathbf{F}_{ii}$, $i \in 4, 5, 6$) need to be added to the trace. The rotationally invariant index measures the stability of the linear equation system (4.5) in the presence of noise.

The adaptation of this quality index would be a straight forward extension of (6.1) for HOT estimation matrices. The original $\mathbf{F}$ was computed from the second order estimation matrix which did not contain a b-factor (see (4.7), the gradient information can be multiplied with b later). If the b-factor is incorporated in the estimation matrix, then the index ν is dependent on the value of this b-factor. Since the estimation matrix for the HOT hierarchy needs to contain more than one b-factor, this index will have problems for inter-model comparison.

6.2.2. Relative Encoding Advantage Factor

The relative encoding advantage factor (REAF) criterion was developed by Hasan et al as extension of the index presented in 6.2.1 to determine the estimation advantage in the diffusion tensor calculations of a given GES over the Icosa scheme with six encoding directions that correspond to the vertices of the regular icosahedron [42]. The Icosa6 scheme is the optimal GES with the minimal required 6 encoding directions (see for

6. Determining The Quality Of Encoding Schemes

example [70]).
$$\text{REAF(GES)} = \frac{6}{N_e} * \frac{\nu(\text{Icosa6})}{\nu(\text{GES})}, \tag{6.2}$$

REAF relates the total variance (ν, see (6.1)) of a given encoding scheme to the total variance of the Icosa scheme and multiplies the result with $6/N_e$ to account for the increase in measurement time caused by the increase in directions. The higher the REAF, the better the encoding scheme (GES) compared to the Icosa scheme with six directions (Icosa6). This index is only applicable for the second order diffusion tensor estimation since the Icosa scheme with six directions cannot be used directly for higher order tensor estimation (see chapter 4).

The optimal schemes for the individual HOT models and tensor orders have not been found, an extension of this index is therefore not trivial. Even if the optimal schemes were known, the index values would not allow an inter-model comparison since the optimal reference schemes would be fixed and not necessarily the same for each model. The reservations toward ν that were presented in section 6.2.1 extend to this extended version.

6.2.3. The Condition Number Of The Estimation Matrix

The condition number, as defined in (5.5), was proposed as a criterion for encoding scheme quality [84]. The lower the condition number, the lower the corresponding upper boundary for the error propagation in the tensor estimation. Batchelor et al showed that the condition number of GESs for the second order diffusion tensor estimation, which are not related to the Icosa scheme, change when the direction set is rotated [10]. They concluded that the rotationally invariant Icosa schemes would be suited best for the second order tensor estimation because of their rotational invariance. In addition, the Icosa schemes all have a condition number of $\sqrt{10}/2 \approx 1.5811$, which corresponds to the optimal theoretical scheme discussed in the introduction of this chapter [10]. The suitability of the condition number as a GES quality measure was questioned previously (see for example [46]). One problem is its rotational dependence. Another one is the interpretation of the condition number as upper boundary, not smallest upper boundary. A low mean condition number does not guarantee a well spread distribution of points on the sphere. This can be seen, for example, in the plot of the Cond GES in Fig.5.7. To represent the variability of the condition number, the GES that is to be evaluated is rotated and the maximal, minimal and mean condition number over all rotations are considered in the classification of the GES [10].

6.2.4. Guaranteed Anisotropic Sensitivity

A different idea is the classification of GES according to how well their encoding directions are spread out (see for example [52, 70]). This is done by taking a look at the angles between the of gradient directions **g**. The guaranteed anisotropic sensitivity (GAS) is a possible measure for the angular distance [52],

$$\text{GAS} = \min(\text{VDP}_{\max}^2 - \text{VDP}_{\min}^2). \tag{6.3}$$

VDP stands for the Vector Dot Product between an average vector and each gradient direction in the scheme. The average vector is the average of a gradient vector and its nearest neighbor. $\text{VDP}_{\max}$ indicates the largest angular distance between an arbitrary direction in the scheme and the nearest neighbor for a given gradient vector. $\text{VDP}_{\max}$ will decrease as the minimal angle between a chosen direction vector and the other directions of the GES, $\theta_{\min}$, increases, which is equivalent to a more regular distribution of gradient directions. It was also suggested to use also the minimal VDP as a quality measure [52].

6.3. Total Variance Of The Second Order Tensor Estimation

The total variance as defined in section 6.2.1 is evaluated for the second order tensor model. All GES families presented in chapter 5 are evaluated with 46 encoding directions. The estimation matrix used in this evaluation does not contain any b-factor. The ro-

Icosa	Ana2	ForceSingle	ForcePairs	Ana1	Cond
0.142	0.143	0.142	0.142	0.147	0.118

Table 6.1.: ν is evaluated for different GES with $N_e = 46$.

tationally invariant results of the evaluation are shown in Tab.6.1. The condition number minimizing GES is clearly favored by this classification method. The force-minimizing GES and the Icosa scheme show similar results for this index. Ana2 performs similar to these schemes whereas Ana1 has a slightly higher total variance.

6.4. Classification By Condition Number For Higher Order Tensor Models

The condition number is a widely used criterion for the determination of GES quality (see also 6.2.3). Opposed to other quality measures, it is directly applicable to all kinds of tensor model estimations, since they all estimate their tensors by solving a linear equation system and the condition number is a property of this system [88]. The degree of rotational variability was used in addition to the mean condition number to determine the quality of a GES because of the rotational variance of this index [10]. A scheme is considered of good quality when the mean condition number is low and the variability of the condition number ([maximal - minimal] condition number) is also low.

For each of the computed encoding schemes, the rotational variance was evaluated by rotating the entire scheme around all three main axes individually and evaluating the

6. Determining The Quality Of Encoding Schemes

condition number of the scheme's estimation matrix for each rotation. The rotation angle varied from 0 to π in steps of 0.001. The comparison of the GES is based on the minimal, maximal and mean condition number.

The rotational variability of the individual GES is illustrated with error bars in the following figures. The ends of the error bars give the minimal and maximal condition number over all evaluations. The differences in rotational variance of the condition number for the encoding schemes which can be seen, for example, in Fig.6.2 illustrate that the mean value of the condition number alone is not a good quality measure.

Second Order Tensor

Some of the here presented schemes were investigated with the condition number as quality measure before (see for example [10, 52]). Here I present a more comprehensive comparison of the condition number for second order tensor estimation matrices. Since the focus in this work is on the higher order tensor models, the results for the second order tensor are only briefly presented. In Fig.6.1 some basic observations can be made:

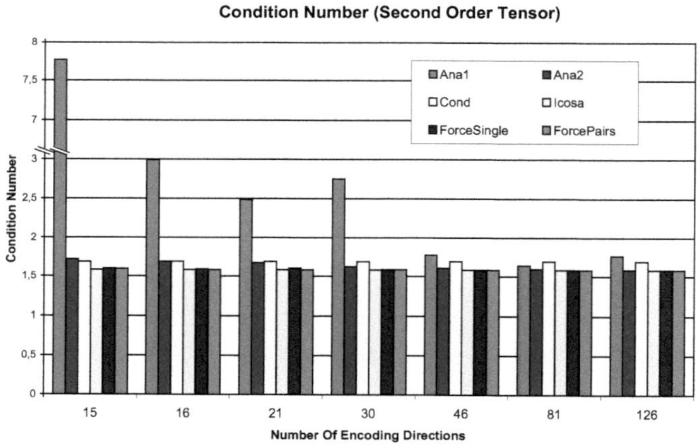

Condition Number (Second Order Tensor)

Figure 6.1.: *The mean condition number evaluation results for the standard second order tensor estimation. The bar for Ana1 with $N_e = 15$ was interrupted to allow the discrimination of the small differences in the condition number for the better performing GES.*

1. The Ana1 GESs require a high N_e ($N_e \geq 46$) to produce an acceptable condition number.

6.4. Classification By Condition Number For Higher Order Tensor Models

2. The mean condition number for the Cond GESs does not improve with increased N_e. It is practically constant.

3. The ForceSingle GES performs similar to ForcePairs for $N_e \geq 30$. For lower N_e the ForcePairs GES performs better.

4. The mean condition numbers of the Icosa GESs and the force-minimizing ones lie close together for all $N_e \geq 15$. This is also true for ForcePairs for lower N_e (not shown here, [10]).

5. The condition number for the Icosa GESs is constant ($\kappa = 1.5811$) for all N_e [10].

A more detailed view of the evaluation that also considers the variability of the condition number, can be obtained from Fig.6.2. The Icosa GESs are rotationally invariant, their

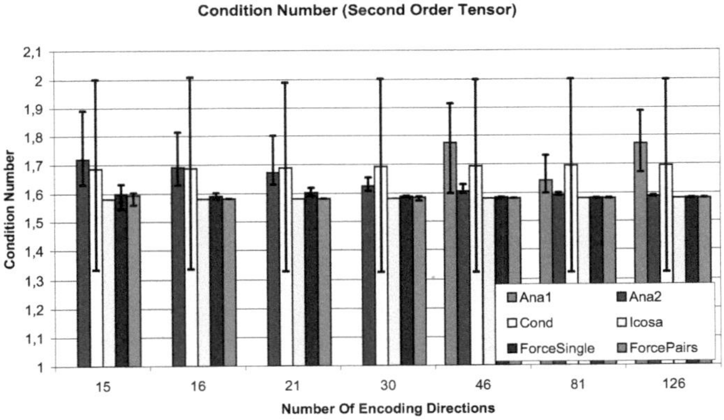

Figure 6.2.: *A more detailed look at the condition number evaluation results for the standard second order tensor estimation previously presented in Fig.6.1. The error bars in this figure give the minimal and maximal condition number encountered in all evaluated rotations. The length of these error bars gives the span of values for the corresponding condition number. Here, the bars for the Ana1 evaluations with N_e = 15, 16, 21, and 30 are omitted to enhance the relatively small differences of the better performing GES.*

condition number is constant. The variability of the condition number for the Cond GESs is almost the same, independent of N_e, for all members of this family. For all other GES a stabilization (reduced variability) is observable with an increase in N_e. A table with all the condition values for the second order tensor estimation is given in the appendix in Tab. A.1.

6. *Determining The Quality Of Encoding Schemes*

Higher Order Tensor Models

Here, I present the results for the single HOT of order four and the HOT hierarchy with maximal order four in detail. This is the tensor order that is required to resolve for example fiber crossing inside heterogeneous voxels. Even higher order evaluations will sharpen the described diffusion profile but voxels for which orders higher than four give necessary additional information are sparse [55]. For the complete higher order evaluation results see appendix A.

The Icosahedral GES For HOT Model Estimations

Batchelor et al recommend the use of the Icosa schemes whose condition number for the estimation of the second order diffusion tensor is rotationally invariant [10]. In my investigation on GES for HOT estimation the Icosa encoding schemes were found to be in general sufficient for the evaluation of the single HOT model up to order eight (45 independent tensor elements) and the HOT hierarchy up to order six (49 independent tensor elements) with at least two b-factors greater zero. Higher tensor orders were not evaluated for this study. However, not all schemes of the Icosa family are fit for the estimation of arbitrary higher order tensor models. The bucky-ball scheme with 30 encoding directions (Icosa30) could only estimate the single HOT model up to order 4, which requires the encoding matrix to have a rank of 15. It did not reach the full rank of 28 needed to estimate the single HOT of order six.

Ne	Ana1	Ana2	Cond	Icosa	ForceSingle	ForcePairs
30	-	172,0	2192,2	-	28134,3	10,3
46	30,2	20,8	81,3	10,2	38,1	10,0
81	14,8	9,9	42,3	10,0	9,9	9,9
126	12,4	9,9	31,2	10,1	9,9	9,9

Table 6.2.: *The mean condition numbers for the GES evaluation of the single HOT model of order 6.*

The mean condition numbers for the estimation matrix of the single HOT model (order six) is given in Tab.6.2. The analytical scheme Ana1 is also not able to generate a full-rank estimation matrix for this tensor model with 30 directions. In fact, the condition number for all GESs but the ForcePairs scheme are very high for $N_e = 30$, these GES should therefore not be used. For $N_e \geq 46$ the Icosa scheme returns reasonably low mean condition numbers. If $N_e \geq 81$, the mean condition number for all but the Cond GES are acceptable but, overall, the ForcePairs GES performs best. The inability of the Icosa GES with 30 directions to produce a full rank estimation matrix for an arbitrary tensor order indicates that the spread of the gradient encoding directions is not the only important GES quality factor. Otherwise, the (mathematically) perfectly equidistributed Icosa scheme with 30 directions [23] should be optimal.

The rotational invariance of the condition number for Icosa encoding schemes [10, 42, 75, 81] cannot be confirmed for higher order tensor evaluations. In my experiments

6.4. Classification By Condition Number For Higher Order Tensor Models

different stabilization behavior for differently constructed icosahedra could be observed. This can be seen in Tab.6.3 and 6.4 where the mean condition number does not always decrease with an increase in N_e. Here, the condition number results are given for the Icosa GES for HOT hierarchy and single HOT of order four. The mean condition number as well as the minimal and maximal condition number over all rotations is given. The observations are also illustrated in Fig.6.4 and 6.6. There is no guaranteed improvement with increased N_e. For example, the variability of the condition number (error bar: minimal and maximal condition number) for the estimation of higher order tensors with 'Icosa30' in Fig.6.4 is higher than the one for 'Icosa21'. The same is true for 'Icosa126' in comparison with 'Icosa81' and for 'Icosa16' compared to 'Icosa15' in Fig.6.6. The schemes, that are based on an even order regular subdivision ('Icosa21' and 'Icosa81') of the regular icosahedron, evaluated here seem to stabilize better for both higher order tensor models than other Icosa GES and therefore are preferable for higher order tensor estimations.

Ne	Icosa		
	max	min	mean
21	499044	484104	489747
30	503308	483747	492999
46	498680	484135	489616
81	490279	484850	486702
126	498055	484188	489392

Table 6.3.: *The condition number results for the Icosa GES evaluation the HOT hierarchy of order four.*

Ne	Icosa		
	max	min	mean
15	5,36	4,09	4,95
16	7,44	6,19	6,86
21	3,85	3,80	3,82
30	3,88	3,82	3,84
46	3,85	3,80	3,82
81	3,80	3,76	3,77
126	3,85	3,79	3,81

Table 6.4.: *The condition number results for the Icosa GES evaluating the single HOT model of order four.*

Further investigations might clarify, whether the differences are systematic and dependent on the construction rules for the individual schemes, which would result in the classification of sub-families inside the group of Icosa schemes. The performance differences between the different Icosa schemes for higher order tensor estimation might

6. Determining The Quality Of Encoding Schemes

indicate systematic differences, which could also affect the second order tensor estimation.

The Condition Number Evaluation For The HOT Hierarchy Model

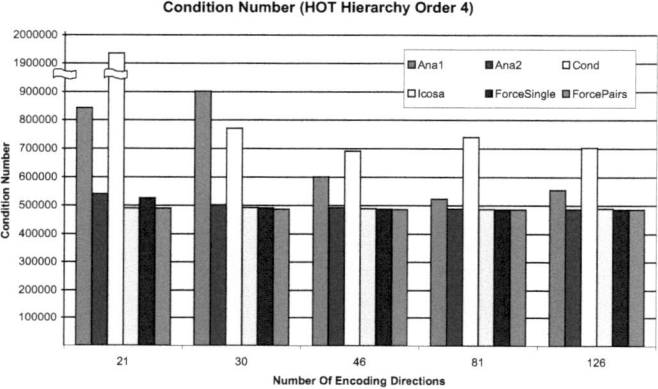

Figure 6.3.: *The mean condition number over all evaluated rotations for the HOT hierarchy. The value for Cond21 is very high and interrupted in this graph to show the small differences of the better performing GES more clearly.*

The results for the HOT hierarchy in Fig.6.3 show that most GES approach a common target condition number of approximately 486000. Only the mean condition number of the Cond GES does not approach this optimum. In fact the mean condition number for this GES does not converge with increasing N_e. This behavior is similar to the observations made in the standard second order tensor condition number evaluation (see Fig.6.2). The Ana1 GES needs larger N_e ($N_e \geq 46$) before the corresponding condition numbers start approaching the target condition number. All other GES whose condition numbers converge toward the target condition number outperform the Ana1 GES. It is therefore rejected. The Ana2 GES shows a low mean condition number, especially for N_e larger 30. The ForceSingle GES performs similar to the ForcePairs GES if the N_e is at least twice the number of independent tensor elements (here 2*21=42). The Icosa and ForcePairs GESs perform best in this evaluation. Their superiority is also observable in the second order tensor evaluation in Fig.6.2. A more detailed look at the best performing GES is taken in Fig.6.4. The error-bars give the value span for the condition number that was observed in the evaluation of the rotational dependence. As expected, the mean condition number of the ForceSingle GES approaches the value for ForcePairs, when N_e larger than twice the minimal required number of directions ($N_e > 42 = 2*21$). The

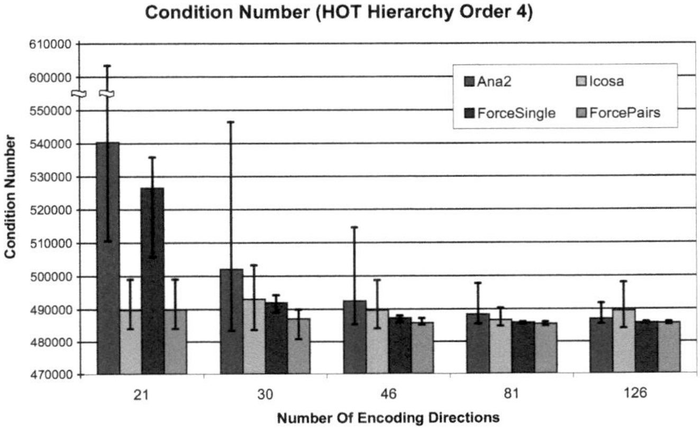

6.4. Classification By Condition Number For Higher Order Tensor Models

Condition Number (HOT Hierarchy Order 4)

Figure 6.4.: *A more detailed comparison of the mean condition number for the HOT hierarchy estimation with the best performing GES is given. In addition to the mean condition number the span of values for the rotational dependent condition numbers is given in the error-bars whose ends correspond to the minimal and maximal condition number over all evaluated rotations. The Y-axis starts at 470000 and is interrupted at 555000 to enhance the differences between the GES.*

mean condition number over all rotations for Ana2 is especially for $N_e > 30$ close to the condition number of Icosa and ForcePairs but Ana2 is always more rotationally variant. Even though the mean condition numbers for the Icosa and ForcePairs GES lie very close together, the ones that correspond to ForcePairs are in general lower. The exact condition number values are given in Tab. A.6 - A.8, in the appendix. The rotational variance for the ForcePairs GES is also considerably lower than for the Icosa GES. ForcePairs is therefore preferable for the HOT hierarchy estimation.

Results From The Condition Number Evaluation For The Single HOT Model

Figure 6.5 shows the mean condition numbers for the single HOT evaluations. The analytical schemes are not able to generate a GES that can estimate the single HOT model of order four with the minimal required N_e of 15. Ana1 can only be used if $N_e > 16$ and is not recommended for $N_e = 21$ because of the relatively high condition number (see Tab.A.4). For $N_e < 30$ for which the tensor estimation with the Ana2 GES would be possible the condition number is too high for this GES to be recommendable (see Tab.A.4). These high condition numbers are not shown in Fig.6.5 so as not to mask small differences in the better performing GES. The Cond GES produces high condition numbers for $N_e < 46$ (see Tab.A.4) which are therefore also omitted from Fig.6.5. Force single

6. Determining The Quality Of Encoding Schemes

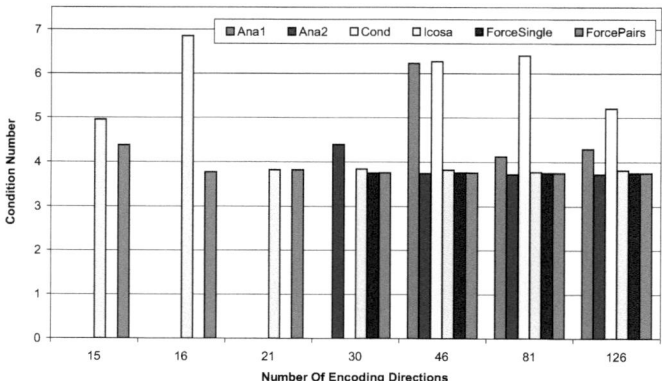

Figure 6.5.: *The mean rotationally dependent condition number for the single HOT model estimation. The comparatively high condition numbers for Cond and Ana1 with $N_e = 15 - 30$ as well as ForceSingle, and Ana2 with $N_e = 15 - 21$ are omitted in this graph to allow the distinction of relatively small differences in the better performing GES.*

has a low condition number for $N_e \geq 30$ (Tab.A.5) but a higher one for low N_e. The results for lower N_e are therefore not shown in Fig.6.5. Only the Icosa and ForcePairs schemes are able to produce estimation matrices with relatively low condition numbers for N_e smaller than 30 (Tab.A.5). For N_e smaller than 21 the ForcePairs GES clearly outperforms the Icosa GES (see also Fig.6.6). For N_e at least twice the minimal required 15 the ForceSingle GES performs similarly to the ForcePairs schemes. This corresponds to the observations made for HOT hierarchy and second order tensor evaluations.

Summary And Discussion

All my condition number evaluations showed that both force-minimizing GESs have similar performance if N_e is larger than twice the number of individual tensor elements. The analytical GESs, especially Ana2, perform well for large N_e, even though they are more dependent on the rotation of the GES. The condition number of the Cond GES does in general neither converge to the target condition number nor stabilize with increasing N_e. The condition number of the Icosa GES is rotationally variant for HOT evaluations. The mean condition number and the variability of the condition number over all evaluated rotations is lower for the ForcePairs GES than for the Icosa scheme for HOT estimation matrices. For the second order tensor the Icosa GES performs slightly better

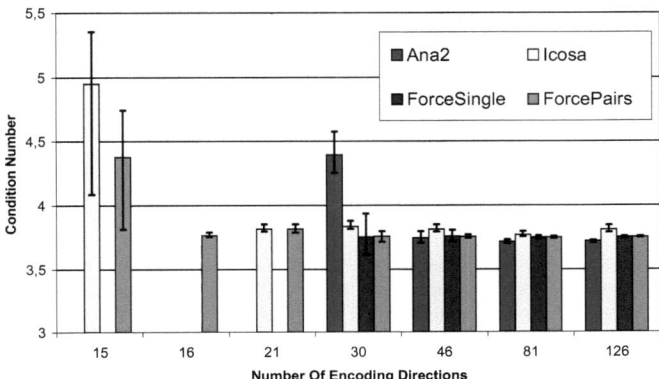

Figure 6.6.: *A more detailed comparison of the best performing GES for the single HOT estimation is given. The bars corresponding to GES with relatively high condition numbers are omitted here to enhance the differences of the GES with lower condition number. To improve the comparability the span of values for the rotationally dependent condition numbers is given in the error-bars which indicate the minimal and maximal condition number over all evaluated rotations.*

than ForcePairs. Overall, the best performing GES is the ForcePairs scheme.

The condition number can be applied to all estimation matrices but the results show significant model-dependent differences hindering cross-tensor-model comparison. Only relative changes can be used for cross-tensor-model evaluations. For a better classification of GES a diffusion-model independent criterion would be desirable.

6.5. Spread Of Directions

The idea to use the distribution of the encoding direction as a measure for GES quality was previously explored, for examples see section 6.2.4. Here, I investigate two distance measures, the angle d_a between the directions **g**:

$$d_a = arccos(\mathbf{g}_i^T \mathbf{g}_j) \tag{6.4}$$

and the electrostatic energy d_e between the projected points on the sphere,

$$d_e = \sum_i \sum_j \frac{1}{|\mathbf{g}_i - \mathbf{g}_j|}. \tag{6.5}$$

6. Determining The Quality Of Encoding Schemes

Both distance measures are stored in $N_e \times N_e$ distance maps for each GES.

The assumption of symmetry of the DWI signal ($S(\mathbf{g}) = S(-\mathbf{g})$; see sections 3.3 and 3.4) make a consideration of the inverse encoding directions on determining the quality of the distributions over the unit sphere necessary. The distance maps were, therefore, investigated for direction sets consisting of the original GESs and their inversions.

Clustering In The Gradient Directions

The complete set of directions for the investigated GES with $N_e = 126$ is given in Fig.6.7. The original directions are given in blue and the inverted ones in red. The directions of the Ana2 GES are well distributed over the unit sphere if only the directions computed by the algorithm (and not their inversions) are taken into account. The points are arranged in a spiral from pole to pole (see Fig.5.4(b)). When the inverse directions ($-\mathbf{g}$) are added to the computed ones ($\mathbf{g}$), the points form two complementary spirals (Fig.6.7(b)) which cross each other several times on their way from one pole to the other. In these regions of crossing, the points are closer to each other than in other regions, they cluster. These clusters obviously reduce the quality of the approximation of equidistribution over the sphere. The other well distributed direction set without inversion is

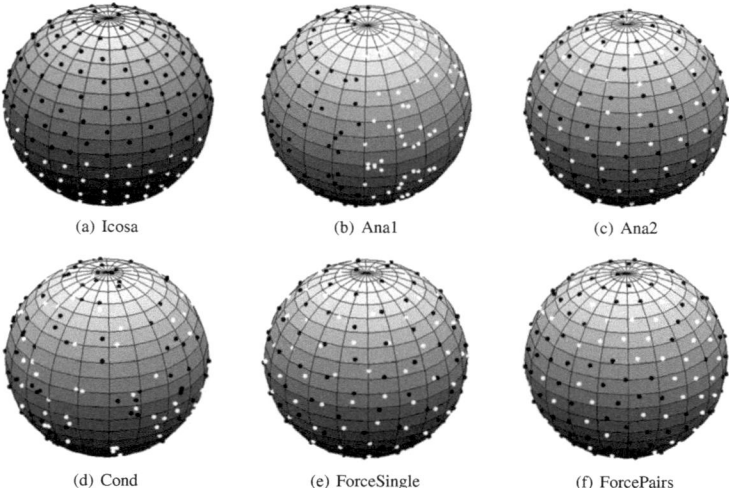

Figure 6.7.: *The distribution of the diffusion encoding directions for the different GES families with $N_e = 126$. The blue dots represent the original directions and the red ones their inversion.*

generated by the ForceSingle GES (Fig.6.7(e)). Since the inverse is not considered in the

6.5. Spread Of Directions

optimization of ForceSingle, the points and the corresponding inversions are arranged in pairs (see Fig.6.8). The pairs draw closer to each other when N_e increases but they generally do not overlap. The Cond and Ana1 GES are not well distributed before the inverse directions are considered. For the irregular distribution of the Cond GES the overall distribution does not improve when the inverse directions are taken into account but usually even more clusters are created with the inverse directions (Fig.6.7(d)). The directions of the Ana1 GES (Fig.6.7(b)) are distributed over a hemisphere, the consideration of the inverse directions, therefore, does not change the relative amount of clustering. The clustering in each hemisphere is equal for Ana1 and the number of points close to the border between the hemispheres is comparably low the amount of additional clustering in these regions is, therefore, also low. The only schemes that have no problem whatsoever with clusters or pairs when the inverse encoding directions are taken into consideration are the ForcePairs (Fig.6.7(f)) and the Icosa GES (Fig.6.7(a)) that arrange their directions under consideration of their inversions.

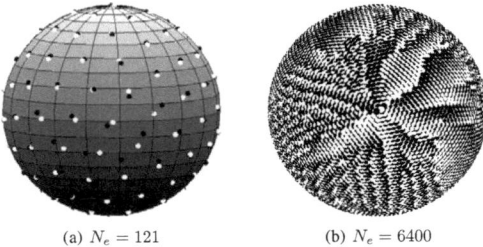

(a) $N_e = 121$ (b) $N_e = 6400$

Figure 6.8.: *The clustering pairs in the ForceSingle GES (gradient directions (in blue) and their inversions (in red)). The direction sets were taken from the homepage of Robert Womersley (http://web.maths.unsw.edu.au/ rsw/sphere/).*

Results From The Angle Investigation

In the angle maps it can be observed that all GESs cover the same interval in the angle histograms in Fig.6.9. The angles are restricted to $\pi/2$, this means angles between the gradient directions greater $\pi/2$ are identified with the corresponding lower angle of their inversion.

Of the evaluated schemes with $N_e = 81$ the ForcePairs GES is the one with the most regular angular distribution. The number of point pairs increase linearly with the angle between them for this GES. This indicates that the distribution of the directions is also very regular. The Icosa GES has the highest number of direction pairs with an angle of approximately $\pi/2$, closely followed by the ForcePairs GES. The Icosa GES has in comparison with ForcePairs two jumps in its histogram. The first is between the first and second angle interval and the second between the last two intervals. These jumps

6. Determining The Quality Of Encoding Schemes

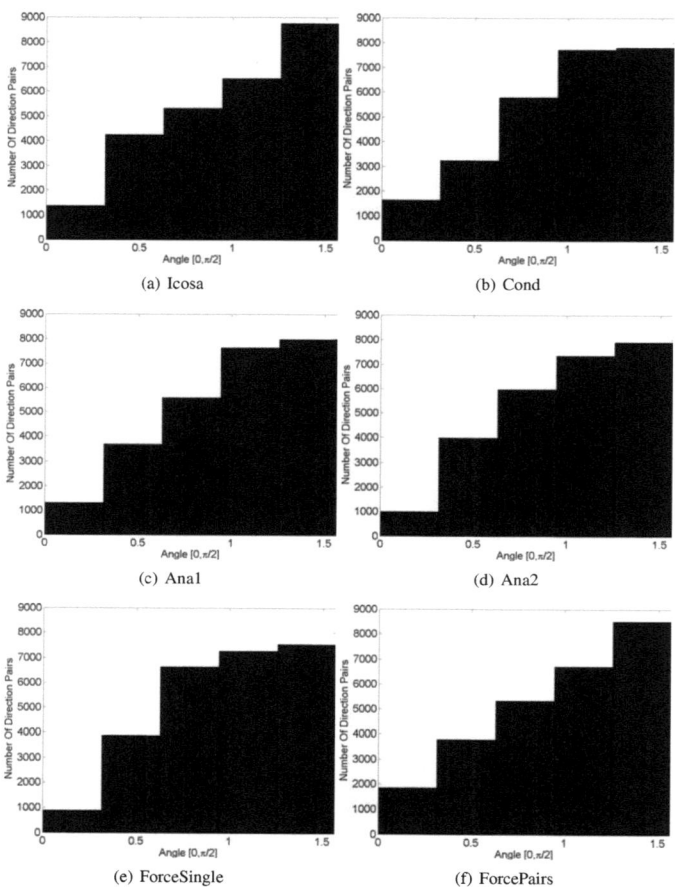

Figure 6.9.: *The histogram of the angular distribution for GESs with $N_e = 81$ for each creation method.*

6.5. Spread Of Directions

allow for the Icosa scheme to have less direction pairs with small angles and more with large angles between them in comparison with the regular ForcePairs distribution. The Cond GES has in comparison with the other GES a large number of pairs with a small angles between them, similar to ForcePairs. In contrast ForceSingle, Ana2 and Ana1 have a comparably low number of direction pairs with small angles. These schemes have similar to the Icosa GES a jump between the first two histogram intervals but the second jump from the Icosa histogram is missing for these schemes. The two histogram intervals corresponding to higher angles ($d_a > \pi/2$) for the ForceSingle and Cond GES contain approximately the same number of point pairs. For the analytical GES the difference in these intervals is also relatively small.

More pairs with a small angle between them might indicate clustering as described in section 6.5 but there is no obvious clustering for ForcePairs (see Fig.6.7). Instead the lower number of large angles between the directions and a high number of point pairs in the center angle interval around $\pi/4$ seems to correspond to the clusters observed in section 6.5. Further distinctions between the GES are not possible with the histogram information. It is, for example, not possible to determine which analytical GES is superior. The ForcePairs and Icosa GES have the largest number of direction pairs with large angles and are therefore, under the assumption that this indicates a low amount of clustering, the best performing GES in this investigation. The Icosa GES has more pairs with large angles and less pairs with small angles. This indicates that this scheme is preferable over the ForcePairs.

A problem with using the angle as classification criterion is that equal angular distribution does not translate into equal distributions of the points on the sphere due to the curvature of the surface. The value of a classification criterion based on the angle between the directions is therefore not clear.

Results From The Electrostatic Energy Investigation

The differences in the electrostatic energy are more prominent (illustrated in Fig.6.10 for $N_e = 81$). Clustering in the directions causes the energy in the individual GES directions to be stronger.

The clusters in the other GESs cause increased energy between the clustered directions. The differences between GESs with and without clusters in the energy-histogram are manifested mainly in a small number of high energy points as can be seen in Fig.6.10. The Cond scheme has in comparison with the Ana2 results a low maximal energy value

Icosa	Cond	Ana1	Ana2	ForceSingle	ForcePairs
0	392	324	192	204	0

Table 6.5.: *Number of point pairs with an energy value greater four.*

but the number of clustering direction pairs ($d_e > 4$) in this GES is the highest in this investigation (see Tab.6.5). The Ana2 GES has the most extreme clusters, producing the largest energy values but the number of clustering points is the lowest one from all

6. Determining The Quality Of Encoding Schemes

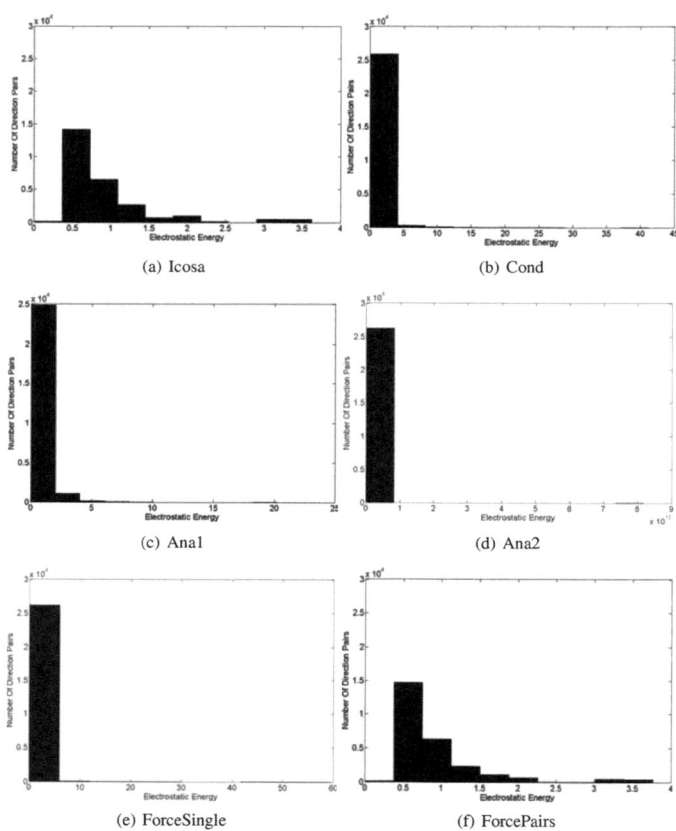

Figure 6.10.: *The electrostatic energy histograms for the GES directions and their inversions.*

6.5. Spread Of Directions

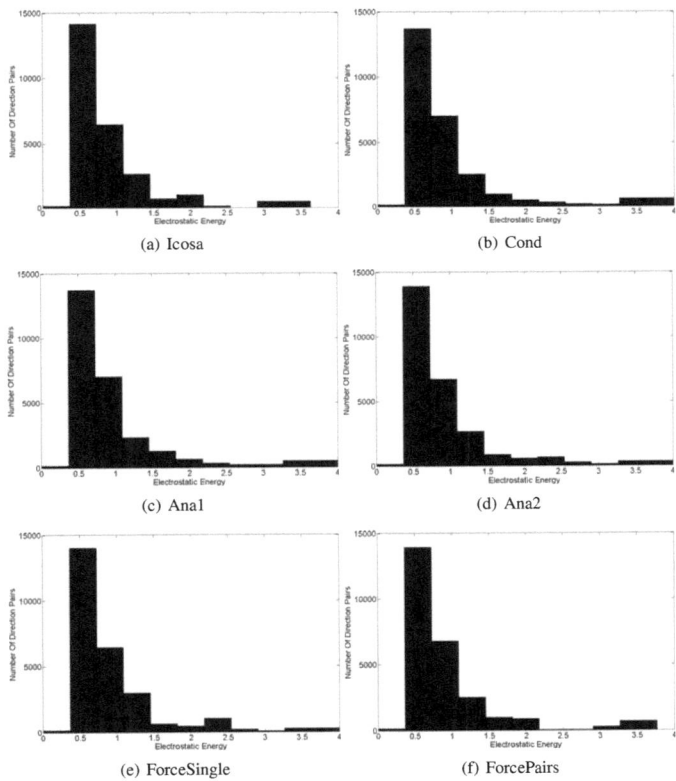

Figure 6.11.: *Details from the electrostatic energy histograms in Fig.6.10 for the GES directions and their inversions.*

clustering GES. The maximal energy value in the Ana1 GES is the lowest one for a clustering GES but the number of clustering points is high in comparison. ForceSingle produces in comparison with the other clustering GES a low number of clustering pairs and a medium maximal energy value.

As first classification criterion I propose the number of clusters. The higher this value the worse the GES. Second is the maximal energy value which should be low. The first criterion clearly disqualifies the Cond GES and possibly also the Ana1 scheme. Ana1 has the lowest maximal energy value of clustering GES in this evaluation and is therefore prefered according to the second proposed criterion. It is not immediately clear if a low maximal energy value outweighs a larger number of clusters. This also complicates the classification of the Ana2 and ForceSingle GES because both schemes produce a similar number of clusters (slightly more for ForceSingle) but the maximal energy values for these GES are very different (far higher for Ana2). It needs to be determined if a high maximal energy value outweighs a lower number of clusters to determine, which of these two GES is favorable over the other.

The comparison of the regions in the histograms corresponding to the energy-interval $[0, 4]$ are very similar for all GES as shown in Fig.6.11. No further classification of the clustering GES is possible from this detailed view.

There are only two types of GES without clusters, the Icosa GESs and the ForcePairs schemes. Both have very similar energy histograms that are restricted to the interval $[0, 4]$ (see Fig.6.10 and 6.12). This shows the relation of both GESs. For six encoding directions, for example, the ForcePairs scheme will approximate the vertices of the regular icosahedron [10]. A distinction in the quality between these two GES from the energy histograms is not possible with this criterion. This is illustrated on the direct comparison of these GES in Fig.6.12. The ForcePairs GES has slightly more direction pairs with low energy [0,0.5] than the Icosa scheme but also slightly more in a higher energy value interval [3.5]. It is not clear which of these aspects weighs stronger and therefore also not clear which GES should be preferred.

For some of the GESs with clusters, such as the analytical schemes and the ForceSingle GES, the spread of the clusters improves with an increase in N_e. The spread of the cluster pairs reduces the number of high energy points in relation to the low energy parts. For the GESs without clusters (icosa and ForcePairs), the relative distribution of the energy values does not change with an increase in encoding directions.

From these results I conclude that the preferable GESs are the Icosa and ForcePairs schemes since they are well distributed and unaffected by the inverse directions. The other schemes all have high energy clusters when the inverse directions are considered in the evaluations.

Summary And Discussion

If the inverse of the gradient encoding directions are taken into account the points on a sphere that are associated with these directions might form clusters. These clusters disturb the equidistribution of the points over the surface of a sphere. The directions Ana1 and Cond show clusters even without the consideration of the inverse directions. The

6.5. Spread Of Directions

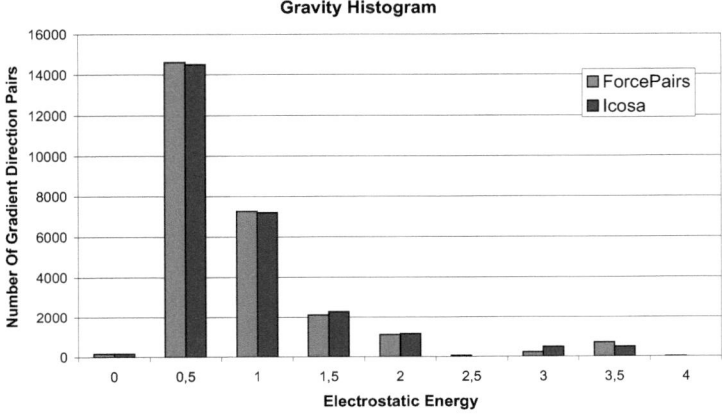

Figure 6.12.: *The energy histograms of the best performing GESs are directly compared.*

directions of the ForceSingle and Ana2 GES cluster with their inversions. The Force-Pairs and Icosa GES are unaffected by clusters because their directions are distributed to approximate an equidistribution over the sphere with their inversions.

The investigation of the angle histogram indicates that the angle could be used to determine clustering in the GES. The Icosa GES is considered best in this investigation followed closely by the ForcePairs GES. The value of quality criteria that are based on the angular distribution of the directions is not clear because equal angular distance cannot be directly translated into equal distance of the points on the surface of a sphere.

My evaluation of the electrostatic energy between the points of the different GES clearly favors the ForcePairs and the Icosa GES over all others. The ForceSingle and Cond GESs produce similar histograms. No clear preference can be given to either one of these two schemes because it is not clear if a larger number of low energy values outweighs the considerably larger absolute energy value for a small number of points. The two analytical GES show comparable performance but the Ana2 scheme performs a little better in comparison.

The energy evaluation clearly shows more differences for the individual types of GES than the investigation of the angle between the direction pairs. This distance measure is therefor preferred over the angular distance. Even though they both favor the same GESs.

6. Determining The Quality Of Encoding Schemes

6.6. Classification By Diffusion Index Estimation Quality

Jones suggested to evaluate an encoding scheme by simulating DTI measurements and assessing the accuracy of diffusion measures derived from the second order tensor estimated from the simulated results [47]. Significant differences in the tensor estimation quality, depending on the orientation of the fiber bundle in the simulation, were discovered. Following the example of Jones I investigated the tensor estimation quality for a larger number of GES by comparison of the noise free tensor with the estimation result from a noisy simulated measurement. The standard deviation of tensor derived diffusion indices such as FA, trace or the principal diffusion direction could be used to determine the estimation quality. Here, I concentrated on the accuracy of the FA computed from the estimated second order tensor as defined in (4.12). This value is of special interest for diagnostic purposes for example in stroke treatment as well as critical for fiber tracking since it is commonly used as tract termination criterion.

For this evaluation I simulated the data by estimating the signal $\hat{S}$ from a given input tensor $\mathbf{D}_{input}$, unweighted signal S_0 and b-factor:

$$\hat{S} = S_0 exp(-\mathbf{B}\mathbf{D}_{input}) \qquad (6.6)$$

This kind of simulation is often used in literature (see for example [53, 47]). Here, two exemplary tensors, one cigar shaped with eigenvalues of 0.0020, 0.0002 and 0.0002 (see Fig.6.13(a)) and one oblate with eigenvalues of 0.0020, 0.0020 and 0.0002 (see Fig.6.13(c)) tensor, were used as input. The elements of the tensors used are given in the appendix C.1. Since the isotropic tensor (ball shaped) has no directionality, the quality of the corresponding estimation does not depend on the orientation of the tensor relative to the GES directions. This case is therefore not considered in the following evaluations.

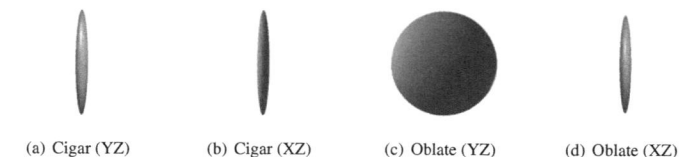

(a) Cigar (YZ) (b) Cigar (XZ) (c) Oblate (YZ) (d) Oblate (XZ)

Figure 6.13.: *The two input tensor used in the simulation (each viewed in YZ and XZ plane).*

To determine the orientation dependent estimation quality the input tensors are rotated in the reference frame. The azimuth angle for the rotation θ ranges from 0 to 2π and the zenith angle ϕ from 0 to π. Both angles are increased in steps of 0.1rad. For each of those 2016 rotations the signal was estimated for the different gradient encoding directions in the individual GES with (6.6). A b-factor of 1000 s/mm^2 was used. Random noise (Noise$_\sigma$) with a mean of zero and standard deviation σ_{noise} is added to this ideal, noise

6.6. Classification By Diffusion Index Estimation Quality

free signal,
$$\sigma_{\text{noise}} = S_0/\text{SNR}. \tag{6.7}$$

If no noise is added to the signal, all GES reconstruct the input tensor perfectly. The aim of this investigation is the evaluation of the noise sensitivity of the tensor estimation depending on the GES used in the signal acquisition, adding noise is therefor necessary. The noise is added according to the following equation (Rician Noise):

$$\hat{S}_{\text{noisy}} = \sqrt{(\text{Re}(S) + \text{Noise}_\sigma)^2 + (\text{Im}(S) + \text{Noise}_\sigma)^2}. \tag{6.8}$$

The signal S is considered complex because the concept of a rotating reference frame as introduced in section 2.1 is transferred to the signal S. To remove the oscillations at the Larmor frequency ω_0 from the signal, that is to transform the signal into the rotating reference frame, the signal needs to be demodulated with ω_0 which results in a split of the actually measured signal into two parts of a complex signal.

The demodulation corresponds to a multiplication of the signal with a sinusoid or cosinusoid with a frequency at or near ω_0 (section 7.3.3 in [36]).

The real part is the signal demodulated with the cosinusoid with frequency ω_0 and the signal in the imaginary part is demodulated with the corresponding sinusoid. The imaginary part of the complex signal $\hat{S}$ contains no significant information for the standard second order tensor and can therefore be assumed to be zero for this case:

$$\hat{S}_{\text{noisy}} = \sqrt{(\text{Re}(S) + \text{Noise}_\sigma)^2 + \text{Noise}_\sigma^2}. \tag{6.9}$$

The noise in both parts of the signal is independent but has the same standard deviation and mean.

The measurements were simulated for several SNR levels (SNR = 5, 10, 15, 20, 25, 30) which are considered typical for DTI acquisitions [47, 53]. To enable a more accurate comparison, the same noise pattern was added to the simulated measurements for the individual GES. 100 repeated measurements with individual noise patterns were simulated for each set of directions and the average FA over 100 repetitions and 2016 rotations of the input tensor was compared. For the individual repetitions, the standard deviation of the FA over all rotations was evaluated. The mean of this value and the span between the maximal and minimal standard deviation over 100 repetitions was also used for a comparison. Even if the mean FA value suggests a good estimation, one can not put a lot of trust in the result if the corresponding standard deviation is large for a certain GES. The GESs were evaluated for $N_e = 6, 10, 15, 16, 21, 30, 46, 81, 126$.

Results Of The FA Reconstruction Accuracy

For comparison, the 'ground truth' was defined to be the noise free tensor from which the simulated signal was computed. The behavior of the different GES were similar for the different SNR levels. The FA values computed from the estimated tensors approach the ground truth with increasing SNR but the relative improvement in the estimation

6. Determining The Quality Of Encoding Schemes

results depending on the number of encoding directions used in the GES was similar independent of the applied noise. The results are therefore exemplarily illustrated on the evaluation for a SNR of 15 in Fig.6.14 and 6.15.

The analytical methods and the ForceSingle scheme were only able to produce GESs for a higher number of encoding directions ($N_e \gg 6$). The schemes with six encoding directions produced by these algorithms resulted in very nearly singular estimation matrices, which is why they should not be used with such low N_e. In this study the two analytical and the ForceSingle GESs are evaluated for $N_e \geq 10$.

The evaluated mean FA for the Cond GES does not converge toward the 'ground truth' value with increasing N_e. Directions are added to this GES in an (almost) random fashion. Therefore, the estimation quality does not improve systematically.

All GES but the Cond scheme will converge toward a common mean FA value with increasing N_e (see Fig.6.14 and 6.15). This target value is lower than the 'ground truth'. This phenomenon can be explained by the added noise. When there is a clear dominance of one eigenvalue (cigar-shaped tensor), very few of the GES directions will show diffusion. For the directions that do not correspond to the dominant diffusion direction (direction of the eigenvector that corresponds to the dominant eigenvalue) no change due to diffusion can be detected. Added noise is very likely to increase the detected change in these directions. This will reduce the dominance of the change caused by actual diffusion and thereby the FA. The same is true for two dominating eigenvalues, especially when they strongly dominate the third.

The Icosa, Ana2 and both force-minimizing GESs estimate the tensors quite accurately. Surprisingly, no clear advantage of the far better distributed ForcePairs or Icosa GES over the other well performing GESs is observable for $N_e \geq 10$ in my evaluation. This indicates that the equidistribution of the directions and their inverse over the sphere is not as important as previously assumed (see for example [47, 49, 76, 84]). This is especially true for a larger number of encoding directions ($N_e \gg 21$). There is not much improvement in the second order tensor estimation quality for the well performing GESs when the number of encoding directions exceeds 21. This result is similar to the results from Jones for the ForcePairs GES [47]. I showed that this is also true for less optimally organized schemes. In Tab.6.6 and 6.7 the results for different GESs with 30 encoding directions are shown. The difference between the Icosa, Ana2 and force-minimizing GESs is only slight. The standard deviation will be further reduced with an increase of encoding directions but the improvement in the FA values is minimal.

The standard deviation of the FA value over all evaluated rotations of the Cond GES is as unpredictable as the corresponding FA (Fig.6.14 and 6.15). The convergence of the mean FA value to the 'ground truth' starts for the Ana1 GES only for $N_e \geq 15$ as illustrated in Fig.6.14 and 6.15. The corresponding standard deviation first increases before it starts decreasing with the other well performing GES for $N_e \geq 16$. This behavior was to be expected since the Ana1 GES is meant for large N_e. The standard deviation of the FA is below 0.04 for $N_e \geq 21$ for the Icosa, Ana2 and force-minimizing GESs. Ana1 is comparable to these GES if $N_e \geq 46$. The standard deviation of the ForceSingle and ForcePairs GESs is very similar for all N_e that allow an evaluation with the ForceSingle GESs ($N_e \gg 6$). This indicates that the advantage of more directions does not directly

6.6. Classification By Diffusion Index Estimation Quality

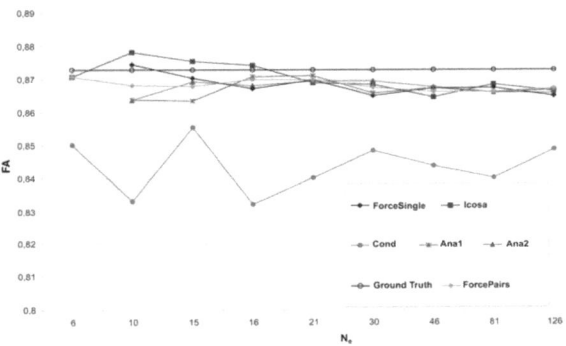

(a) Evaluation of the mean FA values.

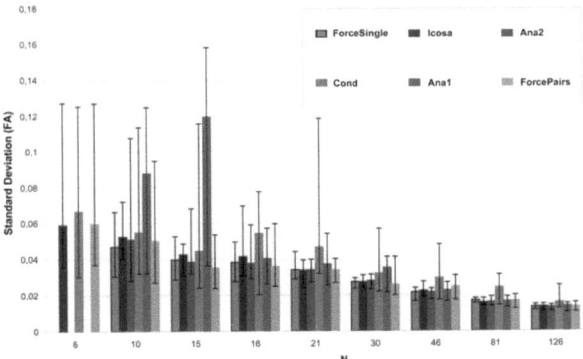

(b) The mean standard deviation of the FA evaluation.

Figure 6.14.: *The evaluation results for a tensor with one dominating eigenvalue (cigar-shaped tensor). The analytical and ForceSingle GESs require larger N_e, and can therefore not be used for the estimation with $N_e = 6$.*

6. Determining The Quality Of Encoding Schemes

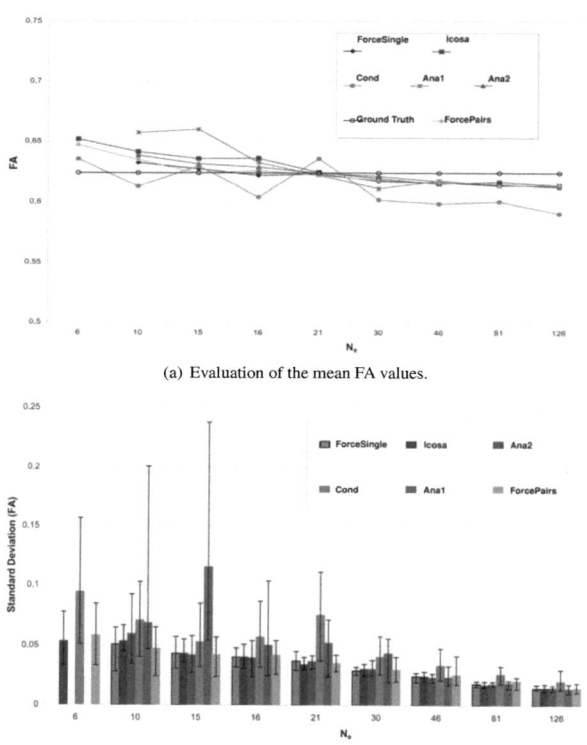

(a) Evaluation of the mean FA values.

(b) The mean standard deviation of the FA evaluation.

Figure 6.15.: *The evaluation results for a tensor with two equally large eigenvalues (oblate tensor). The analytical and ForceSingle GES cannot be used to estimate the second order tensor with $N_e = 6$.*

translate to better sampling of the unit sphere since the sampling of the sphere with ForceSingle for N_e is similar to the sampling with ForcePairs with $N_e/2$.

GES	min(FA)	mean(FA)	max(FA)	std(FA)
Icosa	0.8618	0.8684	0.8763	0.0273
Ana2	0.8605	0.8695	0.8748	0.0279
ForceSingle	0.8620	0.8651	0.8747	0.0273
ForcePairs	0.8602	0.8683	0.8759	0.0260

Table 6.6.: *The tensor estimation results for a cigar shaped tensor for the best performing GESs with* $N_e = 30$.

GES	min(FA)	mean(FA)	max(FA)	std(FA)
Icosa	0.612	0.619	0.629	0.030
Ana2	0.611	0.621	0.627	0.029
ForceSingle	0.610	0.617	0.625	0.028
ForcePairs	0.611	0.620	0.627	0.028

Table 6.7.: *The tensor estimation results for an oblate shaped tensor for the best performing GESs with* $N_e = 30$.

Summary

The Cond GES was found to be ill suited for the second order tensor estimation. Opposed to the other evaluated GES, the results of the Cond evaluation do not converge toward a common FA value. The analytical schemes and the ForceSingle GES require a larger number of encoding directions ($N_e \geq 10$) for the second order tensor evaluation. Ana1 is only comparable in quality to the other GESs if $N_e \geq 46$. The Icosa, Ana2 and both force-minimizing GESs did result in a good quality FA estimation and were equally suited for the second order tensor evaluation with $N_e \geq 21$. There was no obvious advantage of the ForcePairs and Icosa GES over the less well distributed direction sets, which indicates that equidistribution is not the most important quality for a GES.

6.7. Evaluation Of The Signal Representation

Until now no meaningful scalar value similar to FA could be defined for the HOT hierarchy model. Liu et al attempted to define such an diffusion index [Liu07] but could not yet define an index with a clear physical meaning. Without a scalar diffusion index for the HOT hierarchy the *classification by diffusion index estimation quality* that was performed in section 6.6 for the second order tensor model cannot be directly extended to higher order models. For the single HOT model a diffusion index similar to the FA exists

6. Determining The Quality Of Encoding Schemes

[74], but the possible extension of the evaluation from section 6.6 was not investigated here.

A new classification method is proposed that determines the accuracy of the signal representation to quantify the quality of the GES. In this method the estimated signal is used for the comparison instead of a scalar diffusion index. As input the tensors of a HOT hierarchy for a voxel with two orthogonally crossing fibers was chosen. This tensor was estimated from simulated data [57]. The tensor elements are given in C.2. A voxel with orthogonal crossing fibers was chosen for this evaluation because both HOT models should be able to reconstruct such a fiber constellation. Without noise, the input tensor is perfectly reconstructed with the HOT hierarchy model (deviation smaller $1e^{-}13$ for both even order tensors and smaller $1e^{-}7$ for the tensor of order three).

The input tensors were used to estimate the 'ground truth' signal $\hat{S}$ for a given set of directions. The signal is estimated with (6.6). The estimation of the 'ground truth' signal is necessary to be able to evaluate different tensor models. Here, single HOT, HOT hierarchy and the standard second order tensor model are estimated.

To determine the quality of the tensor representation, the signal, corresponding to the estimated tensor, $\hat{S}_R$ is estimated similar to the 'ground truth' signal in (6.6). The estimated signal from the individual tensor models is compared to the 'ground truth' signal ($|\hat{S}_R - \hat{S}|$). The results will show the accuracy of the signal representation of the chosen tensor model and the difference in accuracy of the representation depending on the chosen GES.

To investigate the rotational dependence of the signal representation, the original HOT hierarchy input tensors were rotated in 3D space, before estimating the ground truth signal. A total of 512 rotations were evaluated. The azimuth angle for the rotation θ ranges from 0 to 2π and the zenith angle ϕ from 0 to π. Both angles are increased in steps of 0.2rad.

All tensor models were estimated from data with 10 b-factors ranging for the second order case from 31s/mm^2 to 3092s/mm^2 (as described in section 6.1). The additional b-factors will not contain much new information for the second order tensor and single HOT model estimation but will stabilize the results similarly to averaging of measurements with the same b-factor. The data set with ten b-factors is used in all evaluations for a better comparability of the results.

The following plots show the mean signal deviation (mean error $\bar{\epsilon}$) over all signals normalized with the unweighted signal S_0 for each rotation as defined by

$$\bar{\epsilon} = \frac{1}{s} \sum_{i=1}^{s} \frac{|\hat{S}_R^i - \hat{S}^i|}{S_0}. \tag{6.10}$$

Here, s is the number of acquired signals for each rotation and $\hat{S}^i$ and $\hat{S}_R^i$ are the 'ground truth' signal and the estimated signal for the acquisition i for a given rotation of the GES.

The mean error over all directions $\bar{\epsilon}$ is evaluated for each rotation to investigate the dependence of the accuracy of the signal representation on the tensor orientation relative to the GES directions. The corresponding standard deviation is used to evaluate the variability of the signal representation in the encoding directions for each rotation. A

6.7. Evaluation Of The Signal Representation

GES is considered to be of good quality if the signal accuracy is high (low mean error) and the variation in the signal accuracy is low. The second criterion outweighs the first one because a known error is easier to handle if it is approximately constant.

Noise-Free Evaluation

At first, the accuracy of the signal representation was investigated without noise. The findings are illustrated on the evaluations of a voxel containing two orthogonal crossing fibers for $N_e = 21$.

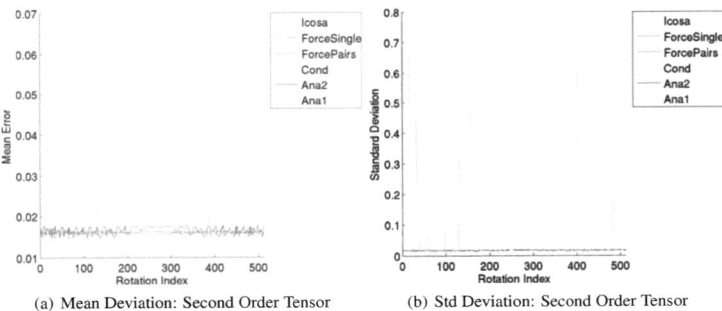

(a) Mean Deviation: Second Order Tensor   (b) Std Deviation: Second Order Tensor

Figure 6.16.: *The evaluation of the accuracy of the signal representation of the second order tensor with 21 directions.*

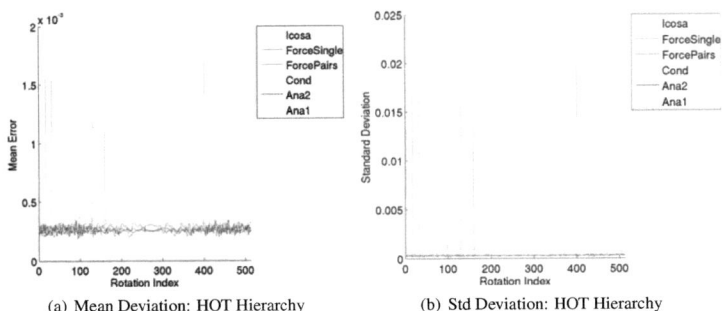

(a) Mean Deviation: HOT Hierarchy   (b) Std Deviation: HOT Hierarchy

Figure 6.17.: *The evaluation of the accuracy of the signal representation of the HOT hierarchy model with 21 directions.*

6. Determining The Quality Of Encoding Schemes

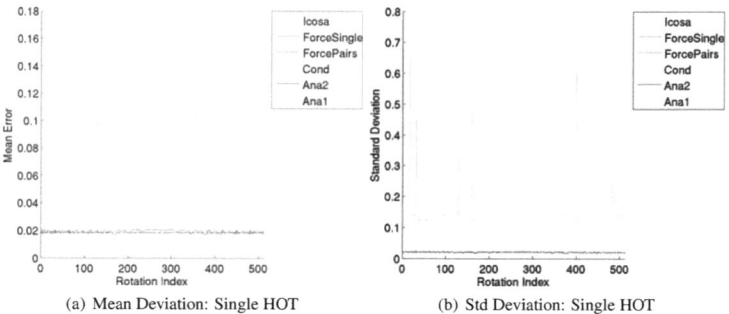

(a) Mean Deviation: Single HOT

(b) Std Deviation: Single HOT

Figure 6.18.: *The evaluation of the accuracy of the signal representation of the single HOT model with 21 directions.*

The differences in signal accuracy for the individual GES in an evaluation without noise can be explained as directional bias in the GESs. A GES prefers orientations on the sphere that are more closely sampled over others. This non-uniform sampling will cause the signal in higher sampled regions to have more effect in the tensor estimation than the signal in lower sampled ones. The tensor representation is therefore biased. This bias will also show in the signal estimated from the tensor representation $\hat{S}_R$ thereby affecting the evaluated signal accuracy. The directional bias is dependent on the spread of the directions and is more clearly observable without noise. In noisy data the mean error not only describes the directional bias but also the noise dependency of the signal accuracy.

GES	Single HOT	Second Order Tensor	HOT Hierarchy
Icosa	0.0185	0.0162	0.0003
ForceSingle	0.0191	0.0168	0.0003
ForcePairs	0.0185	0.0162	0.0003
Cond	0.1610	0.0692	0.0020
Ana2	0.0207	0.0178	0.0003
Ana1	0.0226	0.0186	0.0003

Table 6.8.: *Maximum of the $\bar{\epsilon}$ over all rotations.*

The evaluations show that the signal accuracy is best for the HOT hierarchy (maximal $\bar{\epsilon}$ is 0.002), followed by the second order tensor model (maximal $\bar{\epsilon}$ is 0.07) and the single HOT model (maximal $\bar{\epsilon}$ is 0.2). A complete comparison of the maximal $\bar{\epsilon}$ over all rotations is given in Tab.6.8 for all evaluated GES (with $N_e = 21$) and tensor models. The GES with the largest maximal $\bar{\epsilon}$ over all rotations is always the Cond GES. The Icosa and Force GES produce the smallest maximal $\bar{\epsilon}$ for all tensor models. For the HOT hierarchy all GES but the Cond scheme produce an equally low $\bar{\epsilon}$.

6.7. Evaluation Of The Signal Representation

GES	Single HOT		Second Order Tensor		HOT Hierarchy	
	max	std	max	std	max	std
Icosa	0.0185	0.0000	0.0161	0.0001	2.68E-4	0.15E-4
ForcESinglE	0.0184	0.0002	0.0159	0.0003	2.75E-4	0.31E-4
ForcEPairs	0.0185	0.0000	0.0161	0.0001	2.65E-4	0.14E-4
Cond	0.0962	0.0097	0.0185	0.0063	3.23E-4	1.84E-4
Ana2	0.0192	0.0011	0.0165	0.0008	2.61E-4	0.23E-4
Ana1	0.0185	0.0012	0.0159	0.0010	2.67E-4	0.32E-4

Table 6.9.: *Mean and standard deviation of the $\bar{\epsilon}$ over all rotations.*

The results of this signal accuracy evaluation are shown in Tab.6.9 and in Fig.6.16-6.18. The results for the HOT hierarchy are very accurate. There is, therefore, not much difference in the mean of $\bar{\epsilon}$ over all rotations for the individual GES because $\bar{\epsilon}$ for this tensor model is in general very low as shown in Tab.6.8 and Fig.6.17. The mean of $\bar{\epsilon}$ over all rotations in Tab.6.9 is highest for the Cond GES which also has the highest standard deviation of $\bar{\epsilon}$ and is therefore the most rotational variant scheme for this tensor model. The mean of $\bar{\epsilon}$ over all rotations is very similar for all other GES but the corresponding standard deviation clearly favors the Icosa and ForcePairs schemes.

For the single HOT evaluation the contrast between the Cond GES with a large directional bias and the other GESs is more prominent in Tab.6.9. The Ana2 scheme has the second largest mean $\bar{\epsilon}$ over all rotations and gradient directions. The corresponding standard deviation of $\bar{\epsilon}$ is not low in comparison with, for example, the corresponding standard deviation for the Icosa scheme or the force-minimizing GESs. The Ana2 GES is, therefore, also more rotationally variant than other schemes. The mean $\bar{\epsilon}$ for the Icosa, ForcePairs and Ana1 GESs are the same in this evaluation. The higher standard deviation of $\bar{\epsilon}$ shows the higher rotational variability of the Ana1 scheme in comparison with Icosa and ForcePairs. The mean $\bar{\epsilon}$ for the ForceSingle evaluation is slightly lower than the ones for the Icosa and ForcePairs GESs. The higher standard deviation of $\bar{\epsilon}$ for the ForceSingle evaluation shows that the Icosa and ForcePairs GES are less rotationally variable. The Icosa and ForcePairs GES are therefore preferable because the lower standard deviation of $\bar{\epsilon}$ outweighs the slightly higher mean $\bar{\epsilon}$ over all rotations.

The evaluation of the second order tensor model allows conclusions similar to the ones from the investigation of the single HOT investigation. The contrast between the rotationally more variant GES and the less variant ones is prominent in the plot of the results of the second order tensor evaluation (Fig.6.16).

The difference between the well suitable GES and stronger rotationally dependent schemes is reduced if a larger number of encoding directions is used because all GES show less variability with an increased number of encoding directions. This is illustrated in Fig.6.19 on the example of a crossing voxel evaluated with the ForcePairs GES. As expected, the variability of the signal representation decreases with an increase in the number of encoding directions for all evaluated tensor models. The signal accuracy is less dependent on the orientation of the fibers relative to the GES directions with improved sampling of the sphere by the GES (more directions). The mean $\bar{\epsilon}$ over all

6. Determining The Quality Of Encoding Schemes

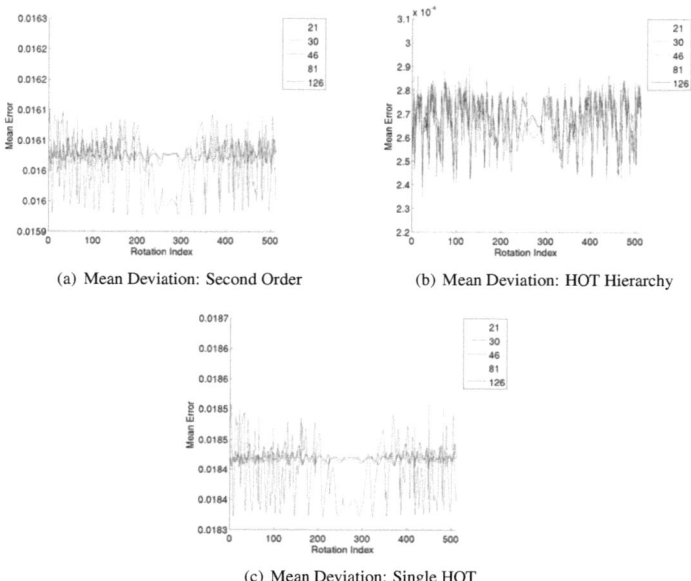

Figure 6.19.: *The signal accuracy for ForcePairs GESs with increasing N_e.*

rotations is approximately constant, independent of the number of encoding directions.

To explain the difference in the signal accuracy, the ADC glyph for the corresponding noise free estimated signals is investigated (see Fig.6.20). The glyphs of the second order tensor model (Fig.6.20(b)) is a disc which is dented in its center (an extension of the peanut shape for a single fiber voxel). The glyph for the HOT hierarchy (Fig.6.20(c)) is, similar to the ADC glyph of the input signal (Fig.6.20(a)), more square than the one for the second order tensor. The glyph for the single HOT model (Fig.6.20(d)) is also square but indented at the sides which pronounces the corners of the glyph. This glyph is also smaller than the ADC glyph corresponding to the input signal. The ADC glyph derived from the second order tensor is larger than the input glyph because it is not square but round. The diagonal that corresponds to the diagonal of the square ADC glyph derived from the input signal is similar in the second order ADC glyph.

6.7. Evaluation Of The Signal Representation

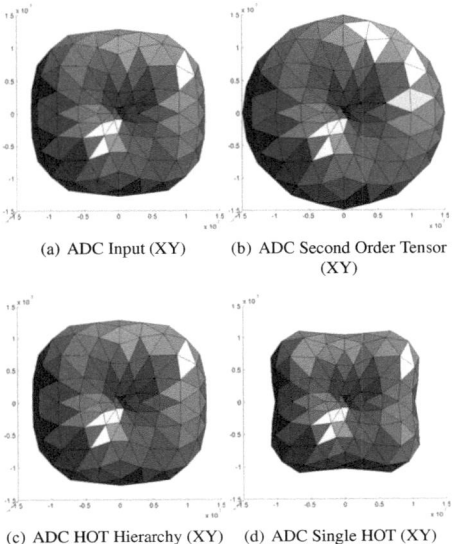

(a) ADC Input (XY) (b) ADC Second Order Tensor (XY)

(c) ADC HOT Hierarchy (XY) (d) ADC Single HOT (XY)

Figure 6.20.: *The ADC glyph corresponding to the different tensor model derived signals for Icosa81 without noise in XY-plane.*

Evaluation With SNR 20

In the second evaluation, Gaussian noise was added to both parts of the complex 'ground truth' signal as shown in (6.8). The resulting SNR for the unweighted signal was 20. The mean error and the corresponding standard deviation are shown in Fig.6.21-6.23. The difference in rotational dependence for the individual GES is not as prominent in the evaluation with noise. Noise will distort the reconstructed signal and therefore blur the small differences between the individual GES. This blurring is especially prominent for the HOT hierarchy evaluation for which all GES except the Cond scheme did perform very good in the evaluation without noise.

The results in Tab.6.10 show that the HOT hierarchy is able to represent the input signal even in noisy data with more accuracy than the other tensor models (maximal $\bar{\epsilon}$ is 0.05). The difference between the maximal $\bar{\epsilon}$ for the individual tensor models is considerably reduced (maximal $\bar{\epsilon}$ for single HOT is 0.2 and for the second order tensor model 0.1). The maximal $\bar{\epsilon}$ for all tensor models are again results from the Cond GES evaluation.

The largest mean $\bar{\epsilon}$ for all tensor models is also result of the investigation of the Cond

6. Determining The Quality Of Encoding Schemes

GES	Single HOT	Second Order Tensor	HOT Hierarchy
Icosa	0.062	0.053	0.048
ForceSingle	0.063	0.058	0.045
ForcePairs	0.062	0.052	0.048
Cond	0.196	0.104	0.054
Ana2	0.064	0.053	0.048
Ana1	0.066	0.053	0.043

Table 6.10.: *Maximum of the mean error over all rotations on noisy data.*

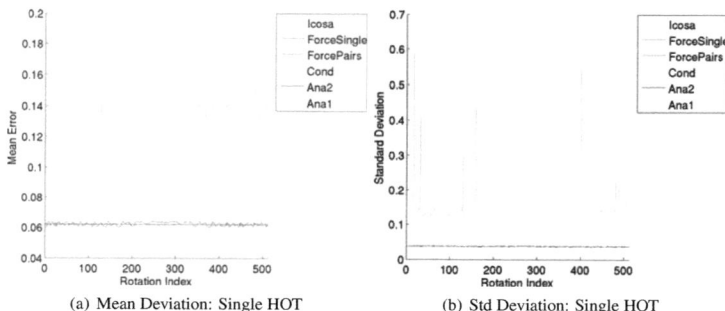

(a) Mean Deviation: Single HOT (b) Std Deviation: Single HOT

Figure 6.21.: *The evaluation of the accuracy of the signal representation of the single HOT model with 21 directions and SNR 20.*

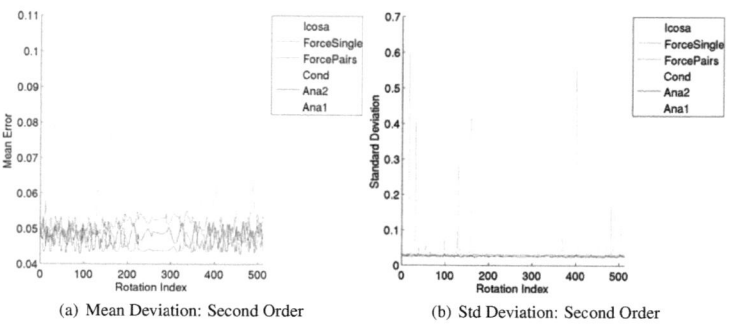

(a) Mean Deviation: Second Order (b) Std Deviation: Second Order

Figure 6.22.: *The evaluation of the accuracy of the signal representation of the second order tensor with 21 directions and SNR 20.*

6.7. Evaluation Of The Signal Representation

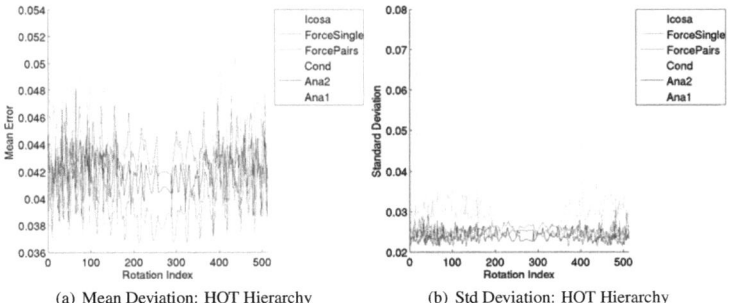

(a) Mean Deviation: HOT Hierarchy   (b) Std Deviation: HOT Hierarchy

Figure 6.23.: *The evaluation of the accuracy of the signal representation of the HOT hierarchy model with 21 directions and SNR 20.*

GES	Single HOT		Second Order Tensor		HOT Hierarchy	
	max	std	max	std	max	std
Icosa	0.062	0.0000	0.049	0.002	0.042	0.0018
ForceSingle	0.062	0.0002	0.051	0.002	0.040	0.0017
ForcePairs	0.062	0.0000	0.047	0.003	0.043	0.0017
Cond	0.135	0.0085	0.055	0.006	0.045	0.0022
Ana2	0.062	0.0010	0.048	0.002	0.042	0.0013
Ana1	0.062	0.0014	0.049	0.003	0.039	0.0014

Table 6.11.: *Mean and standard deviation of $\bar{\epsilon}$ over all rotations on noisy data.*

GES. This largest mean $\bar{\epsilon}$ value corresponds to the largest standard deviation of $\bar{\epsilon}$, similar to the evaluation without noise. The single HOT evaluation clearly shows the increased rotational variability (higher standard deviation of $\bar{\epsilon}$) for the Ana1, Ana2 and ForceSingle GESs in comparison with the ForcePairs and Icosa schemes in Tab.6.11. The high standard deviation of $\bar{\epsilon}$ is considered worse than a low mean $\bar{\epsilon}$ value. Therefore, the ForceSingle and Ana1 GESs are considered worse than the Icosa and ForcePairs schemes. The $\bar{\epsilon}$ values and the standard deviation of the error over all directions for each rotation are plotted in 6.21.

Such a clear distinction is not possible for the other two models in Tab.6.11. This is also illustrated in Fig.6.22 and 6.23. For the second order tensor the ForcePairs investigation did result in the lowest mean $\bar{\epsilon}$ but the larger standard deviation suggests that other GES, for example the ForceSingle scheme, will be preferable. In the HOT hierarchy investigation the analytical schemes are less rotationally dependent than the Icosa and force-minimizing GESs. The results for the individual GES lie close together for these two models in the evaluation without noise. Therefore, the performance loss for the Icosa and ForcePairs GES here is attributed to noise which blurs the results for the individual GES.

6. Determining The Quality Of Encoding Schemes

The improvement in signal accuracy with an increase in N_e is more prominent in the investigation with noise as illustrated in Fig.6.24. For the HOT hierarchy model (Fig.6.24(b)) not only a decrease in variability but also a decrease in $\bar{\epsilon}$ is observable with an increase in N_e. For the single HOT model the variability does decrease with an increase in N_e but the mean $\bar{\epsilon}$ is approximately constant for all GES (mean $\bar{\epsilon}$ is 0.06). For the second order tensor the scheme with $N_e = 30$ has a higher mean $\bar{\epsilon}$ value than the evaluation with $N_e = 21$ which decreases again for higher N_e. The standard deviation for this tensor model evaluation does always decrease with an increased N_e.

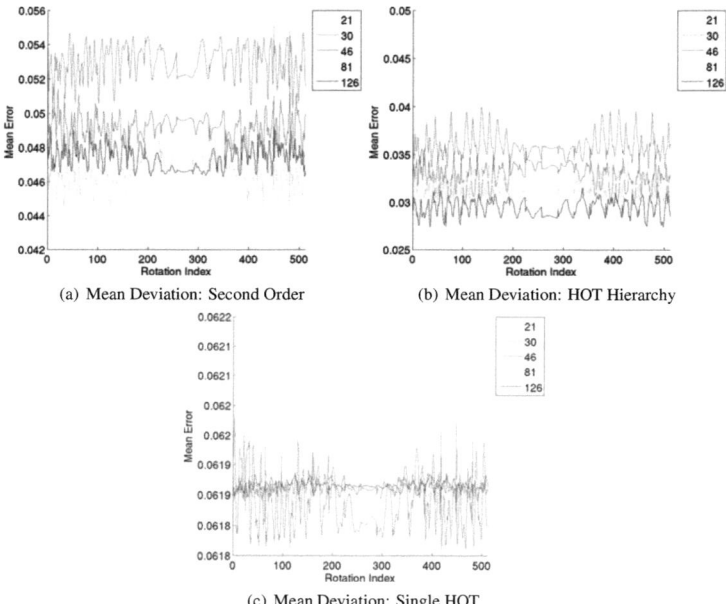

(a) Mean Deviation: Second Order

(b) Mean Deviation: HOT Hierarchy

(c) Mean Deviation: Single HOT

Figure 6.24.: *The signal accuracy for ForcePairs GESs with increasing N_e on noisy data.*

Summary

The Cond GES was found to be disadvantageous for all evaluated tensor models. Also, the Ana1, Ana2 and ForceSingle schemes could be discarded because the other schemes give a better signal fit in the evaluation without noise.

The signal fit is best for the HOT hierarchy model (max $\bar{\epsilon}$ is 0.05 in the evaluation of the noisy signal) and worst for the single HOT diffusion representation (max $\bar{\epsilon}$ is 0.2 in the investigation on the noisy signal). An increase in directions will reduce the rotational variability of the signal fit (standard deviation of $\bar{e}$), independent of the added noise.

6.8. Summary And Discussion Of The GES Evaluations

Most evaluated quality measures did recommend the Icosa and Force Pairs GESs and discarded the Cond scheme. This is in accordance with the second order tensor evaluations in literature (see for example [10, 47]). The only evaluation that did prefer the Cond GES was the total variance (section 6.3). The Cond GES is universally rejected in the literature and by the other classification methods evaluated here. The total variance is, therefore, rejected as quality measure for GESs. With this disqualification of the total variance the extended version REAF (section 6.2.2) is also rejected because all reservations toward the total variance also apply to REAF.

Even if the total variance did not prefer the Cond GES, an inter model comparison of the results would be problematic because of the b-factor dependence of this quality index. The different models require different b-factors and the HOT hierarchy even introduces a new b-factor model with the b-factors of higher order. This will render the results very individual for each model and the applied b-factors. The inter model comparison is also problematic for REAF because the optimal GES for the individual model are not known. The basis for the encoding advantage therefore needs to be determined first to be able to evaluate this quality measure.

The condition number as quality index is also not usable for an inter model comparison because this value varies dramatically depending on the estimation matrix of the model. Opposed to REAF this quality index is directly applicable for all here evaluated tensor models.

The results from the second order tensor condition number evaluation (see section 6.4, Fig.6.1) show that the condition number was much lower (similar to the one for Force-Pairs) for ForceSingle when N_e was at least twice the number of independent elements in the tensor model that was to be estimated.

The preferred GESs in this evaluation were Icosa and ForcePairs. For higher order tensors evaluations the condition number is not constant for the Icosa GES but rotationally variant similar to the condition numbers for other GES for all tensor models. The mean condition number of ForcePairs GES is for higher order tensor models lower and less rotationally variant than the one for Icosa GES. The ForcePairs GES is therefore preferred.

The analytical schemes did perform well for large N_e, especially for Ana1 the N_e need to be very large ($N_e \geq 46$) for this scheme to be comparable to the other well performing ones. The Ana2 GES is performing similarly to the Icosa and ForcePairs GES for $N_e \geq 30$. The mean condition number of the Cond GES does not improve systematically with an increase in N_e, it stays comparably high. This scheme is therefore rejected.

Differences in the behavior of the condition number for the Icosa scheme that are dependent on the construction of the directions were observable for the higher order

6. Determining The Quality Of Encoding Schemes

tensor evaluations (section 6.4). The hypothesis of a systematic difference in the Icosa schemes could not be confirmed in my extensive second order tensor diffusion index estimation quality evaluation (section 6.6) but the differences for this simple diffusion model could be too small for relatively high N_e to be observable.

The Cond GES is the only scheme for which the FA value in the evaluation in section 6.6 does not converge. This GES is rejected because, especially, for the cigar shaped tensor in Fig.6.14, the FA value reconstructed by this scheme is not close to the 'ground truth'. Ana1, Ana2 and ForceSingle require $N_e \geq 10$ to be able to estimate the second order tensor model but then do perform well. All GES but the Cond scheme perform similarly well for $N_e \geq 21$. Icosa and ForcePairs are preferred because they can also handle $N_e \leq 10$ well.

The classification by diffusion index estimation quality (section 6.6), contradicts the results for the GAS index (see section 6.2.4) published in [52], the Icosa16 does not provide better results than Icosa15. The GAS index was therefore not considered here.

The hypothesis that GES that have approximately equidistributed directions over the sphere perform better than others could not be confirmed in the second order tensor evaluation presented in section 6.6. There was no difference between the Icosa and ForcePairs GESs and the other evaluated schemes observable for higher N_e.

The consideration of the inverse gradient directions in the evaluation of the spread of the encoding directions show the reason for some phenomena observed in the other evaluations of the GES. All GES but the Icosa and ForcePairs schemes contain direction clusters if the inversion is taken into account. With an increase in N_e the clustering pairs in ForceSingle and Ana2 grow closer and the clusters loose importance. The clusters can explain why the ForceSingle GES behaves similar to ForcePairs with $N_e/2$ in the condition number evaluation (section 6.4). The clustering pairs of directions and their inversions lie close together. The inverse encoding directions, therefore, do not improve the coverage of the whole sphere, opposed to the inversions in ForcePairs. If N_e is larger than twice the number of independent tensor elements the less optimal sampling of the sphere with ForceSingle has no grave effect on the GES quality. The Cond and Ana1 schemes cluster even before the inverted directions are considered. The clustering with inverse directions does not affect Ana1 as dramatically as the Cond GES because the directions of this scheme are distributed on a hemisphere, additional clusters might only occur on the border of the hemisphere. The clustering with inverse directions in the Cond scheme is as random as the initial directional distribution.

The quality measures that are based solely on the encoding directions (angle and electrostatic energy in section 6.5) could find the well performing criteria but could not clearly distinguish between the individual clustering GES. The value of an angle based quality measure is not clear since a well angular distributed scheme does not necessarily approximate an equidistribution of the points on a sphere surface. The angle quality measure is therefore disregarded. The energy index (section 6.5) is able to show more differences between the non-optimal GES than the angle. Even so the classifications of the other schemes differ considerably from the other evaluations, especially for the ForceSingle GES which is considered comparable to the preferred GESs for large N_e in the condition number evaluation (section 6.4), but does not perform well in the energy

6.8. Summary And Discussion Of The GES Evaluations

evaluation (section 6.5). The energy index is therefore also disregarded.

The evaluation of the signal accuracy (section 6.7) is able to support all findings from previous classification attempts that were not discarded or disregarded. This quality measure can clearly show an advantage of the force-minimizing and icosahedral GES over the analytical ones which was not as clear previously. This method is the only one that can be directly applied to all tensor models and possibly also to other signal representations (for example SHD or the multi-tensor model) to allow a direct comparison. The evaluation of the signal representation is therefore the most promising of the GES quality measures evaluated here. To determine the full capability of this quality measure an optimal set of input tensors needs to be defined. In addition to a comparison of GES a comparison of the evaluated tensor models is also possible with this quality measure.

The accuracy of the signal fit is dependent on the number of b-factors that are used and will improve with an increase in b-factors. For better comparability I did evaluate all tensor models on a dataset with 10 b-factors. This high number of b-factors is not suitable for practical application but it is not to be expected that the relative behavior of the individual GES will depend much on the number of b-factors. The comparison should therefore not depend on the individual choice of b-factors. The optimal number and choice of b-factors for the HOT hierarchy is still undetermined. This is a topic for future investigations. The actual accuracy might decrease with the number of b-factors but it is to be expected that the fit will remain superior to the other two models if evaluated on the same data set, with the same b-factors.

The signal accuracy can only be evaluated for specific input tensors. It needs to be determined if the relative accuracy between the different GES changes depending on the input tensor. A change was not observable in my investigations but another set of input tensors might provide one. The optimal set of input tensors needed to classify the tensor estimation quality of a GES needs to be determined.

The new classification by signal accuracy is able to clearly identify the Cond GES as worst GES. Also a distinction between ForceSingle, the analytical GESs and the better performing Icosa and ForcePairs GESs is possible with and without noise. The difference in the evaluation without noise can be explained by direction encoding bias. Especially clustering GES prefer some diffusion directions (the clustering ones) over others and, thereby, introduce a directional bias to the signal.

The ForcePairs and Icosa GES are generally the schemes with highest quality. From the condition number results for HOT models (section 6.4) show an advantage of ForcePairs for HOT estimations. This and the fact that Icosa is not able to produce an approximate equidistribution over the sphere with an arbitrary number of encoding directions, led me to the conclusion that the ForcePairs GES is the best GES for general use. This scheme is closely followed by the Icosa GES. Ana2 shows also reasonably good performance but since the other two GES clearly outperform this scheme for lower N_e it is disregarded. The Ana1 GES is discarded the same as the Cond scheme, even though the Ana1 scheme is the better of these two.

7. Fiber Tracking

An important question in the investigation of the brain concerns the connectivity of individual gray matter (GM) regions. The neurons in the GM are connected with each other and other parts of the organism by axons that form the so called white matter (WM; for more detail on the anatomy of the brain see section 3.1). The understanding of brain connectivity in itself is an interesting subject for scientific pursuit but the connectivity information of individual patients could also be used for diagnostic purposes. Connectivity evaluations are for example used to monitor and predict the course of degenerating neuronal diseases such as Alzheimers. Information on connectivity can also be important for surgery planning. The surgeon can base his decision on where to cut in brain tumor removal not only on his own experience but also on the connectivity information which tells him where important fiber pathways most likely pass the tumor.

Before DTI was available there were only invasive means to investigate brain connectivity. In nonhuman primates, for example, connectivity between anatomically separate brain regions could be detected by injecting tracers into one region and observing the transport of these tracers postmortem. This technique can identify a connection between individual synapses but this type of study is not feasible on living human subjects. The postmortem preparation of the brain that does not disturb the fiber pathways is also not trivial. This is especially true for fibers that do not run in parallel with the cuts in the prepared brain. Since the brains of different species differ significantly, the tracer results from animal studies cannot be applied to humans directly.

The human brain could, previous to the discovery of DTI, only be investigated postmortem by gross dissection or histological staining [15]. The information that can be gained from human postmortem studies is limited, since WM tracts start deteriorating directly after death. All the above methods are not suitable for diagnostic purposes. Degeneration studies on patients with documented brain lesions are a kind of in-vivo study on humans. These studies can in general not be transferred to other patients, because lesions are highly individual.

The discovery of DTI enabled non-invasive in vivo studies on human subjects. In early experiments it was observed that water diffusion in fibrous tissue, such as brain or muscle, is stronger in the direction of the fibers then perpendicular to them [12]. It is assumed that the diffusion is hindered by the fibers' membranes. From the diffusion information one can therefore infer the direction of the fibers contained in the subject. The reconstruction of whole fiber pathways from this information is termed fiber tracking. At the moment fiber tracking is the only non-invasive method for the investigation of GM connectivity in living human subjects.

A lot of different methods were proposed for the reconstruction of the fiber tracts from the discrete voxel-based diffusion information. Some of the more established methods are presented in the section 7.1.

7.1. Established Tracking Methods

Several fiber tracking methods are known from literature. The most established and oldest approach is the so called streamline method, which is based on line propagation. This method will be presented in more detail in section 7.1.1. The problems of this basic tracking method are discussed in 7.1.1.2 and some alternative front propagating tracking approaches are introduced in short in section 7.1.2. All tracking is inaccurate because of measurement noise and PVE. The reconstructed fibers therefore may deviate from the actual anatomy and are therefore referred to as 'fiber tracts'. The inaccuracy led to the development of fiber tracking methods that determine the probability that a reconstruction corresponds to an actual tract. The most prominent probabilistic fiber tracking methods are presented in 7.1.3.

7.1.1. Streamline Tracking

The oldest and most commonly used family of tracking algorithms for neuronal pathways is based on line propagation, so called *streamline* techniques ([8], [20], [61] and [68]). Streamline tracking (SLT) is based on the assumption that all fiber populations in a voxel are aligned along a single orientation. Under this assumption the principal eigenvector which belongs to the largest eigenvalue of the diffusion tensor corresponds to the direction the diffusion is strongest in the evaluated voxel. To reconstruct a fiber pathway, one simply has to follow these principal eigenvectors from voxel to voxel. Since the direction of the principal eigenvector **d** is ambiguous, the tracking is started in both possible directions (**d** and **-d**) from the origin of reconstruction. The line propagation in the reconstruction has to be terminated at some point because of the finite length of the fibers [69]. Without formal criteria the propagation may continue infinitely.

7.1.1.1. Tract Termination

The most intuitive criterion for tract termination is an anisotropy threshold. In voxels with low anisotropy, such as for example voxels containing brain gray matter, no coherent tract orientation is reconstructible and the principal eigenvector direction will be more sensitive to noise errors. The fractional anisotropy in brain gray matter is typically lower 0.2, hence an anisotropy threshold of 0.2 is a popular choice for this termination criterion (see for example [69]). The tract is terminated when the anisotropy in the current voxel is below the chosen threshold.

Anatomically plausible tracts are usually smooth. The assumption of Gaussian diffusion inside a voxel prohibits sharp turns in the fiber orientation. A threshold for the angle between the principle eigenvectors in two successive voxels is generally used as a

7. Fiber Tracking

smoothness criterion to prohibit sharp turns in the tract which would violate this assumption [69]. Sharp turns that would violate the smoothness criterion might be caused by a sharp U-turn in a fiber that cannot be resolved in the given data resolution (voxel size) or by fiber crossing where the fiber that corresponds to the reconstructed tract is dominated by a larger fiber bundle. In the case of crossing fibers the smoothness criterion is especially important to avoid false tract reconstruction.

7.1.1.2. Known Problems

The SLT algorithm has some drawbacks. It is relatively sensitive towards noise in the acquired data because it uses only the principal eigenvector for the tract reconstruction. All measured data is to some extend subject to measurement noise. The noise sensitivity of fiber tracking methods is therefore an important issue which needs to be taken into account when interpreting the tracking results. For example, the actual principal eigenvector and the vector corresponding to the second largest eigenvalue could switch places in the measured tensor because of noise. This exchange would cause the reconstruction to follow the wrong vector leading to false results. In a voxel with low anisotropy the diffusion represented by a compromised tensor could become even lower, which could lead to a violation of the FA threshold and an abrupt stop in the reconstruction of the tract. In addition, errors along the reconstructed path are accumulated, causing even slight errors to result in faulty reconstructions. The error increases with the tract length.

Another drawback of the SLT algorithm is the fact that it only follows one fiber tract on leaving a voxel, thereby providing a one-on-one mapping between voxels, rendering the reconstruction of tract branching impossible. A fixed step length in the reconstruction will cause problems reconstructing curving fiber pathways accurately [61]. The tract is not able to follow the curvature accurately. The reconstructed tract will deviate more from the path of the curving fiber with each step of the reconstruction. This is illustrated with the tract of red arrows in Fig.7.1 which deviates from the fiber (long black arrow) that is to be reconstructed.

To improve the reconstruction especially for curving tracts the FACT (fiber assignment by continuous tracking) algorithm was developed [68]. FACT works on a continuous vector field instead of a discrete one. Each reconstruction step starts in the point the reconstructed tract enters the next voxel. This results in a more accurate reconstruction of the pathways since the reconstructed trajectory is more flexible. As shown in the example in Fig.7.1, the tract (marked squares) reconstructed with FACT in the right illustration follows the fiber pathway (long black arrow) accurately.

To further improve tracking, especially in the presence of curving tracts, the reconstruction along a tract can be propagated with small steps of predefined size [8, 20]. The direction of the next step is then determined by distance-averaging the principal eigenvector orientations of the surrounding voxels. This will result in an even smoother tract. In more rigorous approaches averaged diffusion tensors are used to determine the fiber orientation instead of averaged eigenvectors. The directions computed from averaged tensors are more accurate because the effects of noise on the eigenvector (as discussed in the beginning of this section) can be reduced in comparison with the averaged eigenvec-

7.1. Established Tracking Methods

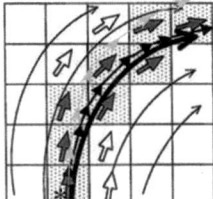

Figure 7.1.: *The thick dark arrow represents the fiber that is to be reconstructed. The tract reconstructed with steps of equal size (in light gray) deviates from the fiber that is to be reconstructed. It can be seen that the reconstruction on a continuous vector field (thin black arrows) track the path of the fiber more accurately. The graphic was adapted from [68].*

tor approach.

The limitations in the measurement accuracy allow fibers with a diameter of 1-10 μm to cross, kiss or branch inside of a voxel which has usually a side length of one to several millimeters. The estimated diffusion tensor in such a voxel represents the averaged signal of all individual fibers (partial voluming effect, see section 2.5.2) because only the total diffusion inside the voxel's boundaries can be measured. The different fiber orientations a voxel contains can therefore not be distinguished in the second order diffusion tensor used to commonly evaluate DTI data. This presents a general problem for fiber reconstruction because the primary eigenvector of a tensor representing the averaged signal does not necessarily correspond to the orientation of a real fiber. Therefore, reconstruction will be inaccurate or fail completely in voxels containing more than one fiber orientation. These partial voluming effects may also result in less anisotropic tensors, for example in regions of fiber crossing as illustrated in Fig.7.2, causing premature termination of the tract reconstruction. A way to adapting the basic algorithm to overcome some of these PVE related problems has been suggested for example in [28]. Here, the algorithm continues tracking in the neighborhood of the voxel the previous reconstruction terminated in because of low anisotropy. If the low anisotropy is confined to a small region, it can be bridged by this type of neighborhood tracking.

Any tracking result also depends on the choice of the initial reconstruction seed, the so called region of interest (ROI). This makes the results hard to reproduce since the manual definition of a ROI on a given anatomical landmark differs from investigator to investigator and even for one investigator from day to day and acquisition to acquisition. The image contrast can differ in each measurement rendering accurate ROI placement in multiple data sets very difficult. Differences in the ROI used as origin for the fiber tracking result in sometimes drastically different reconstructed tracts because slight variations in the ROI might include neighboring fibers into the tracking results or exclude fibers on the border of the anatomy. To avoid this problem a so-called multi-ROI approach was

7. Fiber Tracking

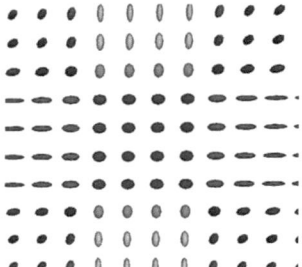

Figure 7.2.: *The effect of tensor averaging is illustrated by two crossing fibers. On the fibers the diffusion glyphs are cigar shaped. In the intersection of the fiber pathways the shape gets more spherical, that is less anisotropic. The fiber running from left to right (red) is slightly dominating the top-down (green) pathway. This plot was generated with the TensorViewer of the MedInria software package [29].*

suggested [20, 87]. This method first performs a brute force streamline reconstruction, each voxel in the dataset is a seed voxel for a streamline reconstruction. The results are filtered by the application of one or multiple ROIs (see Fig.7.3). This filtering approach allows the use of a relatively large ROI for a crude selection of the anatomy that is to be investigated (see Fig.7.3(b)). This crude selection is then refined with additional ROIs as illustrated in Fig.7.3(c).

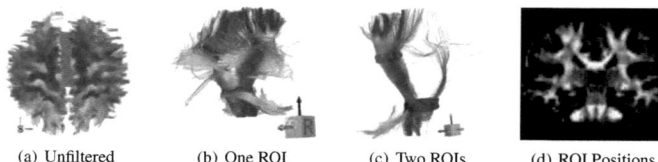

(a) Unfiltered   (b) One ROI   (c) Two ROIs   (d) ROI Positions

Figure 7.3.: *Tract reconstruction with 'brute force' (a) and filtering of the results with one (b) or multiple ROIs (c). The positions of the ROIs are marked on an axial FA slice in (d).*

7.1.2. Front Propagating Methods

An alternative to the streamline tracking approach that in its basic form reconstructs only one-on-one connections between voxels uses front propagating methods to establish fiber connections [18, 44, 56, 78, 79]. These methods use the fast marching technique from level set theory [83] to propagate fronts that evolve at a rate determined by the diffusion

7.1. Established Tracking Methods

information. Some examples for front propagators are the principal eigenvector of the diffusion tensor [78, 79] and a probability measure for the primary diffusion direction [18]. When a point in the evaluated data set is passed over by the propagating front, the so called 'time of arrival' (TOA) is stored in a map. From this TOA map, paths can be reconstructed with a gradient descend through the data set. The descend starts from the outermost front and tracks back toward the origin of the front propagation. The position of the front is determined in each iteration step. To do so the speed of the front propagation $speed_F$ needs to be calculated in each candidate. One possible definition of the speed of the propagated front for the easiest case that uses the principal eigenvector λ_1 in the propagation is given by:

$$speed_F(\mathbf{r}) = FA(\mathbf{r}) * |\lambda_1(\mathbf{r})n(\mathbf{r})|, \tag{7.1}$$

$n(\mathbf{r})$ is the normal of the front in candidate $\mathbf{r}$. $FA(\mathbf{r})$ is the anisotropy in $\mathbf{r}$. The front is propagated fastest in regions where n and λ_1 are collinear. A candidate is a point neighboring the actual diffusion front that might be passed over by the front in the actual iteration (gray in Fig.97). A candidate is passed over by the front if the arrival time $T(\mathbf{r})$

$$T(\mathbf{r}) = T(\mathbf{r}') + \frac{|\mathbf{r} - \mathbf{r}'|}{speed_F(\mathbf{r})} \tag{7.2}$$

is smallest for all candidates. $\mathbf{r}'$ is a point on the actual front. The dependence of the front propagation on $speed_F$ ensures a rapid propagation in the dominant diffusion direction λ_1. This propagation is also illustrated in Fig.7.4. This reconstruction method allows for

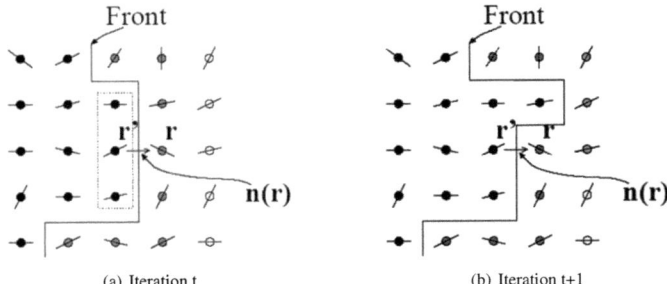

Figure 7.4.: *Illustration of the front propagation with the fast-marching technique. The front propagation depends on the normal of the front ($n(\mathbf{r})$) and the principal eigenvectors in the individual voxels (lines through the points). This figures are adapted from [78].*

tract branching, which presents a problem for the standard SLT. Branching fibers reunite automatically in the backtracking reconstruction. It is also able to continue tracking

7. Fiber Tracking

in regions with low anisotropy that would prevent SLT reconstruction. These methods return a possibly large number of fiber tracts. It is therefore advisable to assess the probability that a reconstructed tract corresponds to an actual anatomical neuronal fiber bundle to select the important tracts from the reconstruction. Some probability measures for this purpose are presented in the next section.

7.1.3. Probabilistic Tracking

All fiber tracking algorithms make the assumption that the acquired data is not affected by noise. This is of course unrealistic in data sets resulting from actual measurements. Each reconstruction step on the tract is therefore subject to a certain amount of uncertainty because of noise in the data. Similar to the error, the uncertainty will accumulate with each step of the reconstruction. This means uncertainty will increase with the distance from the initial ROI. An additional source of uncertainty in the reconstruction is the incomplete modeling of the diffusion signal with for example the simple second order tensor model. The inaccuracy can be illustrated when tracking results starting in point A and ending in B are compared with the results starting in B. The tracking is not bijective, i.e. the results from the second experiment will not necessarily return to A. To classify the reliability of the reconstruction, the probability of the reconstructed tract can be specified, for example with the methods presented in [13, 18, 45]). The so generated probability maps can be used to discard reconstructions with low probability. The methods for the construction of these probability maps are numerous. Some more prominent methods are presented in more detail in the following paragraphs. Note that probabilistic tracking methods only quantify the support of an connection between two points based on the evaluated data. They do not answer the question whether a connection exists at all in real life.

A local method that characterizes the accuracy of a voxel's diffusion tensor representation was introduced by Jones in [45]. This approach uses 'bootstrapping' [27] to generate a large number of DTI data sets from a given number of data acquisitions. Bootstrapping is a method from statistics that creates 'new data sets', the so-called bootstrap samples, by randomly combining the voxel data from several individual measurements. These random estimations of the DTI data sets can be used to generate voxelwise statistics. A special local probability measure was proposed by Jones that describes the uncertainty of the primary eigenvector of the diffusion tensor (in [45] called '95 percent confidence angle') by evaluating a voxelwise statistic over the principal eigenvectors from all bootstrapping samples. The 'cone of uncertainty' was proposed as visualization for this statistic The orientation of this glyph corresponds to the mean principal eigenvector direction over all bootstrap samples. A cones whose cross section corresponds to the confidence angle is used to illustrate the possible deviation from this mean. The slimmer the cone, the more confidence can be put into the accuracy of the tensor representation. This method gives the local uncertainty of the diffusion representation.

A visualization method for local probability values along reconstructed fibers is the use of stream tubes [95] or hyper streamlines [24]. Both are glyphs that add local diffusion information to the principal eigenvector direction coded in the reconstructed streamline.

7.1. Established Tracking Methods

The cross sections of such a tract representation usually give information on the two smaller eigenvectors of the local diffusion tensors. The previously mentioned 'cone of uncertainty' could also be combined with these tract-glyphs to visualize the local uncertainty along the tract. This visualization method allows local assessment of the probability only. The probability of a connection between point A and a distant point B cannot be directly determined from this local information.

To determine the probability of an actual connection between two points A and B a global measure of connectivity needs to be defined (for examples see [13, 77]). If there is no uncertainty in the local fiber directions, the probability of a connection is equal to one if SLT can reconstruct a fiber tract starting in A and reaching B. The probability is zero otherwise. To accommodate the uncertainty in the diffusion direction several diffusion direction samples are randomly generated from the local probability density functions (PDFs) with Monte Carlo methods, similarly to the previously presented bootstrapping approach. The diffusion direction samples might deviate from principal diffusion direction, depending on the PDF. The SLT algorithm is started in A for each sample. By counting the amount of so reconstructed tracts passing through the individual voxels and dividing this number with the total number of tracking evaluations, each voxel can be assigned a probability value for its connection with the starting point A. By adjusting the termination criteria for the tracking algorithm as suggested in [13, 77], a connectivity measure can even be computed for regions that would not have been reached by standard tracking, such as brain gray matter. The probability values are used to separate the highly improbable reconstructions from more realistic tracts if the thresholds for the tract termination are lowered. An example evaluation is given in Fig.7.5. In Fig.7.5(a) the probability values are given for each slice and laid over the corresponding FA maps (Fig.7.5(b) gives a close-up of the slice containing the single voxel ROI). This map shows a connection of the marked ROI with relatively distant regions. The probability decreases with the distance from this ROI. It is hard to gather usable 3D information from this set of probability slides. A 3D visualization of the probability values with high probability values is given in Fig.7.5(c).

Ehricke et al use local PDFs to determine regions of fiber crossing or branching [28]. Where ordinary SLT reconstructions would terminate, secondary tracts are reconstructed in neighboring voxels and connected with the previously terminated tract pieces. The so produced tracts are enriched with an index that determines the probability that an arbitrary point on a reconstructed tract is actually connected to the tracking seed. This global probability measure weights the value of the local PDF with the probability of the previously reconstructed path. This guarantees that the probability will decrease along the reconstructed tract, which corresponds to the observation that tracking errors accumulate during the tracking process (see 7.1.1.2). Opposed to the previously discussed methods, this approach does not establish its probability values by statistics over the results of repeated SLT reconstructions. The probability value in this method is only dependent on the local PDF and the probability of the previous reconstruction.

7. Fiber Tracking

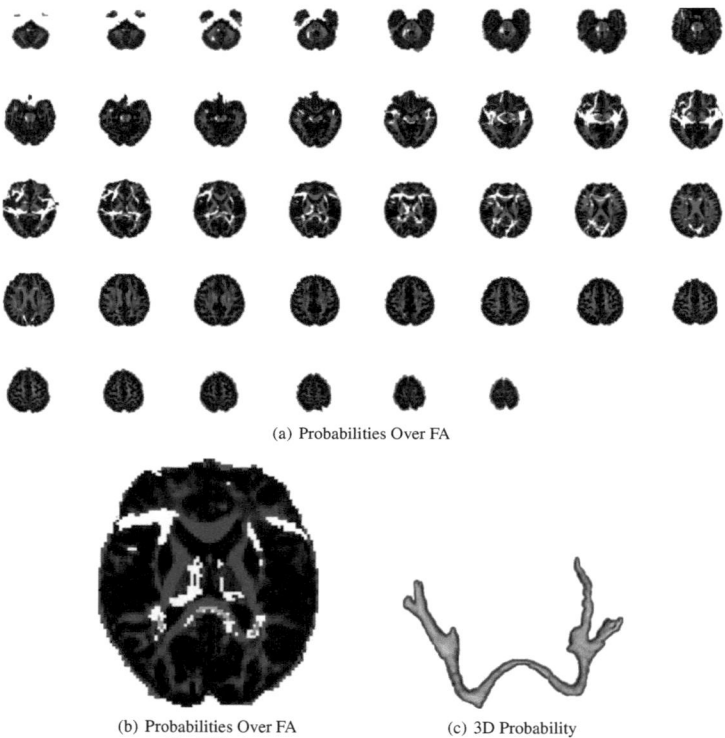

(a) Probabilities Over FA

(b) Probabilities Over FA
(Seed Slice)

(c) 3D Probability

Figure 7.5.: *The results of a probabilistic tracking method (overlayed on a FA map), generated with the FSL/FDT [31] software package.*

8. Diffusion Simulation Based Tracking

The idea of investigating neuronal connectivity by simulating anisotropic diffusion has been explored previously [11, 33, 51]. Similar to the fast marching methods described in section 7.1.2, this approach is based on expanding fronts. Diffusion Simulation Based Tracking (DSBT) generates expanding fronts by simulating the spread of a virtual concentration peak. The simulation numerically solves the diffusion equation which describes a natural physical phenomenon. The propagation of the front is determined by the measured diffusion tensor information, which reflects the anatomy of the measured subject. This approach exploits the whole tensor information of the evaluated neighborhood and is accordingly more robust against noise and more reliable in the reconstruction, opposed to the front propagating fast-marching techniques that most often use the principal eigenvector for the front propagation.

8.1. The Basic Algorithm

The DSBT algorithm reconstructs trajectories based on the idea that a simulated diffusion will be stronger in directions corresponding to the course of neuronal fibers. This is similar to the assumption underlying all DTI and DWI measurements. According to this assumption the maximal spread of the front of the simulated diffusion can be assumed to correspond to the course of the actual neuronal fibers. The algorithm consists of three major steps. First, a virtual concentration peak is generated in a user defined region of interest. This concentration then dispenses during a simulation process. Iso-concentration surfaces are extracted from the simulation results and termed 'diffusion fronts'. From these fronts, the fiber tracts are reconstructed. The tracts need to satisfy termination criteria similar to the ones used in SLT reconstructions (see section 7.1.1.1) to exclude anatomically implausible tracts.

In [51] this basic idea was implemented by successive simulation of diffusion for a short fixed time period on coherent points, i.e. points satisfying the termination criteria. The coherent points on the diffusion front of a simulation are future simulation seed points. Two succeeding points (one on the diffusion front and the other the simulation origin) are connected with a straight line. This way the fiber tracts are built up recursively. One of the main advantages of DSBT over SLT methods is the intrinsic handling of fiber branching. The backtracking reconstruction that connects the outermost diffusion front with the simulation origin allows for fibers to unite on the way. This is a common trait of all front propagating methods.

8. Diffusion Simulation Based Tracking

My new DSBT method evaluates the simulated diffusion over several time steps. Simply bridging the distance between the simulation seed and the points on the outermost diffusion front similar to the approach in [51] would result in tracts that might lack in curving details. To avoid this, a time of arrival (TOA) map is used in the reconstruction. TOA maps have been used successfully in previously published front propagating fiber tracking methods (see section 7.1.2). In the TOA map the time of flooding, that is the time the diffusion front reaches a point, is stored for each point in the evaluated data set. With a gradient descend on this TOA map the fiber tracts are reconstructed. The individual steps of the algorithm are discussed in more detail in the following sections.

For the illustration of the DSBT algorithm, here, only single voxel ROIs are used in the explanations and evaluations. An extension to ROIs that encompass multiple voxels is straight forward. DSBT, as described here, is evaluated successively for each voxel in the ROI to compute the complete reconstruction.

8.2. The Simulation

In the simulation step the diffusion equation (see also section 3.2),

$$\frac{\partial C}{\partial t} = \nabla \cdot (\mathbf{D}\nabla C), \tag{8.1}$$

is solved numerically. Here C is the user defined particle concentration, t is a fixed constant time step and $\mathbf{D}$ is the diffusion tensor computed from the measurements. C is high in a selected region of interest (ROI) and (approximately) zero elsewhere. The definition of the initial concentration peak C ($t = 0$) is discussed in more detail in the following section. The simulation is performed for several time steps to propagate the diffusion front over the evaluated region.

8.2.1. Initialization Of The Concentration Peak

Before the simulation can begin the particle concentration needs to be initialized for all grid points. The initialization is a peak over a user defined ROI. The initial peak should fit the user defined ROI as well as possible. This means the sides of the peak should be as steep as possible for an accurate reconstruction. Flatter sides might, especially for small ROIs, result in artificial enlargement of the ROI. This is illustrated in Fig.8.1 for a single-voxel ROI. The dirac-like initialization on the left has a concentration value greater zero only in the user defined ROI. All reconstructed tracts are therefore connected with this ROI directly. The diamond shape in the top view of this initialization (see Fig.8.1(c)) is a result of the interpolation for the visualization between the high concentration value in the center of the peak and the surrounding background with a concentration of zero. The bell-shaped Gaussian initialization on the right has a wider base. The reconstructed tracts originating from an enlarged ROI will not necessarily be connected to the original user defined ROI, which would in the here discussed example be the center point of Fig.8.1. This renders the tracking results less accurate.

8.2. The Simulation

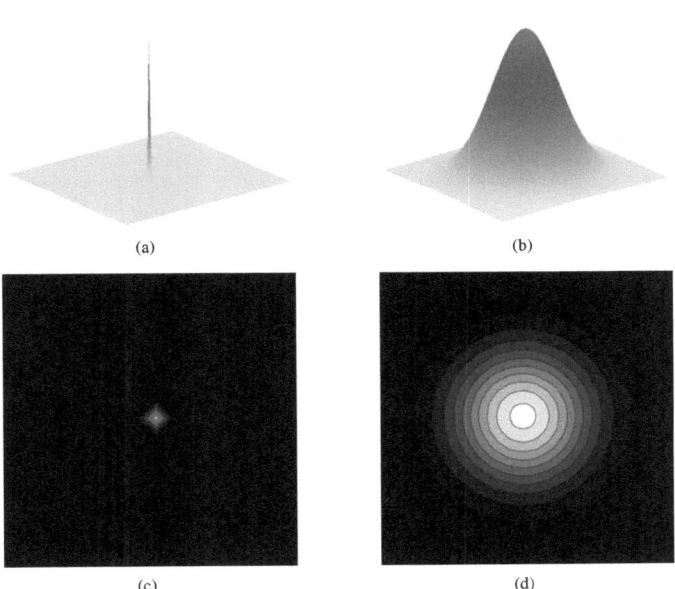

Figure 8.1.: *The flattening of the sides of the initial peak will enlarge the ROI that is used in tracking. This is illustrated in the comparison of an Dirac-like peak (left) with a Gaussian peak (right). In the lower row of images the size of the projected ROI is illustrated. The size of the ROI corresponding to the Gaussian peak corresponds to the outermost ring in (d). The size of the ROI in (c) is exactly one voxel.*

8. Diffusion Simulation Based Tracking

The ideal dirac-like initialization is not as smooth as the bell-shaped one. This can cause problems in the simulation process which are discussed later on in section 8.5

8.2.2. Implementation

For the computation of the simulation two possibilities were explored. First, FEMLAB [19] which is based on Matlab (The MathWorks, Inc.; Version 7.1.0.246 (R14) Service Pack 3), was used. Second, the SG2 library [1] developed in the research group 'Simulation in Technology' at the University of Heidelberg, Germany (directed by Prof. Dr. G. Wittum) was employed. Both methods evaluate the simulated diffusion on a discrete data grid.

FEMLAB: Femlab uses a finite elements method (FEM) to approximate the exact solution of the partial differential equation (PDE that describes the diffusion process (8.1)). The FEMLAB software allows easy definition of the initial concentration and uses well tested algorithms. A problem with this software is the handling of dirac-like initializations. This type of initialization is not continuous and can therefore not be handled by the FEMLAB solver directly. The solver smooths the initialization prior to the first simulation step, which results in subzero concentration values at the base of the concentration peak. These subzero regions will decrease with each simulation step but they still present problems in the computation of the TOA maps because they cause a non-monotone decrease in the concentration values. The resulting effects will be more clear when the TOA map has been introduced in more detail in the following section. Subzero regions could be avoided by smoothing the initial peak, flattening the peak's sides. This is equal to smoothing the edges of the ROI which leads to artificial enlargement of the ROI as discussed before, especially with single voxel ROIs.

SG2: The SG2 [1] solver used in the final implementation was customized for this project by Dr. D. Logashenko (Steinbeis Research Center 936, Oelbronn-Duerrn, Germany). The equation (8.1) is solved numerically with an initial concentration of

$$C_{\text{init}}(\mathbf{r}) = \begin{cases} 1 & \text{if } \mathbf{r} \in \text{ROI} \\ 0 & \text{else} \end{cases} \tag{8.2}$$

as illustrated in Fig.8.1(a). On the boundaries of the evaluated volume a stationary concentration value of zero is chosen. To compute a solution of the diffusion problem (8.1) that is comparable to the analytical solution, the PDE needs to be discretized on a (finer) grid. The numerical solution will converge towards the analytical one as the discretization control volume size that corresponds to the voxel size on the discretization grid approaches zero.

The discretization methods used here are the implicit Euler method on the primary grid which corresponds to the input data grid, in time and the vertex-centered finite-volume (FV) method (also referred to as box method, for example in [35]) for the secondary

8.2. The Simulation

grid of control volumes in space. The control volume grid is defined so that each data point is the centroid of a rectangular control volume. The sides of the control volume are equal to the spatial distance of the data points on the primary (discretization) grid in the individual directions, this means they are equal to the voxel size in the data acquisition. The FV method computes the concentration change that is the sum of all incoming and outgoing particle flux to determine the new concentration values ($C_{new} = C_{old} +$ flux). The particle flux needs to be evaluated for this control volume with the flux function:

$$\mathbf{J} = -\mathbf{D}\nabla C. \tag{8.3}$$

It is sufficient to only evaluate the flux through the faces of the control volume.

$$\mathbf{F}_f(C) = \int_f \mathbf{J} \cdot \mathbf{n}\, df_i, \tag{8.4}$$

$\mathbf{F}_f(C)$ is the flux through the control volume face f, f_i are the points on this face and $\mathbf{n}$ is the corresponding outer normal vector. The integral in (8.4) is approximated by

$$\mathbf{F}_f(C) = |f|(\mathbf{J}_{fc} \cdot \mathbf{n}), \tag{8.5}$$

with $\mathbf{J}_{fc}$ the flux function evaluated in the centroid of the control volume face f and $|f|$ the size of the face. The required concentration gradients are computed with finite differences as illustrated for the top face in a 2D example in (8.6) and Fig.8.2. The concentration gradient in the opaque green star in Fig.8.2 can be computed with

$$\frac{\partial C}{\partial y} = \frac{C(\mathbf{r}_{(0,1)}) - C(\mathbf{r}_{(0,0)})}{h_y} \tag{8.6}$$

$$\frac{\partial C}{\partial x} = \frac{1}{2}\left(\frac{C(\mathbf{r}_{(1,0)}) - C(\mathbf{r}_{(0,0)})}{h_x} + \frac{C(\mathbf{r}_{(0,1)}) - C(\mathbf{r}_{(-1,1)})}{h_x}\right). \tag{8.7}$$

The position $\mathbf{r}_{(0,0)}$ is the center of the control volume, $\mathbf{r}_{(1,0)}$ its neighbor to the right and $\mathbf{r}_{(0,1)}$ the data point on top. h_x is the length of the control volume in X-direction, h_y the one in Y-direction. These equations are illustrated in Fig.8.2. The blue points are the data points $\mathbf{r}$ that are used to compute the derivatives. The derivative in Y-direction is computed from the central difference of the two blue neighboring points $\mathbf{r}_{(0,0)}$ and $\mathbf{r}_{(0,1)}$. In X-direction the derivative is the mean of two differences (non-opaque green stars). The formula in (8.7) should only be used if the off-diagonal element in the diffusion tensor (D_{xy}) is smaller zero. Otherwise, the points $\mathbf{r}_{(0,0)}$, $\mathbf{r}_{(0,1)}$, $\mathbf{r}_{(1,1)}$ and $\mathbf{r}_{(-1,0)}$ are used in the differences.

The large linear equation system which results from the discretization is solved with BiCGSTAB [5] iterations, preconditioned with the geometric multi-grid method with ILU smoothers. This choice of solver allows reasonably fast, efficient, and stable computation. Note that the matrix of the discretized linear system can be asymmetric because of changing anisotropy of the data set. Therefore, we apply BiCGStab instead of CG to solve the system. The multigrid method [37] is used to further speed up the computation.

8. Diffusion Simulation Based Tracking

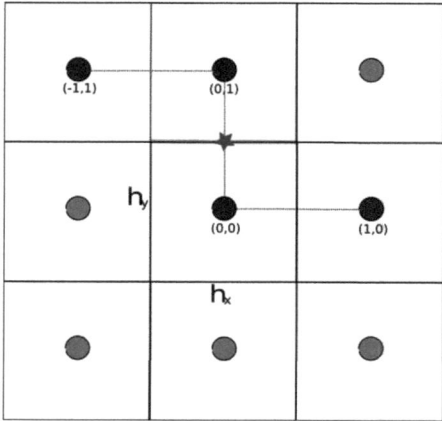

Figure 8.2.: *The approximation of the flux with finite differences is illustrated.*

This C++ based SG2-simulation is not only more than ten times faster than the FEM-LAB simulation but also allows the use of dirac-like initializations without artifacts. SG2 does not produce non-monotone, subzero concentration values. To compensate for small artifacts caused by the non-continuous dirac-like initialization, the results of the first simulation step are discarded.

8.3. The TOA Map

From the simulation results a TOA map is constructed. This map contains the time stamp corresponding to the simulation step in which each individual point was reached by the diffusion front. The detection of the diffusion front is of special interest in the TOA map construction and will therefore be discussed in more detail. The front detection in TOA map based DSBT is slightly more complicated than in other front-propagating fiber tracking techniques (see Fig.8.3). In the fast-marching approach, for example, there is no data point in between two adjacent fronts. Opposed to this, the diffusion front in DSBT can pass over multiple points in the same direction during a simulation step. In the DSBT approach proposed in [51] the front is classified by a constant threshold. This is sufficient in this case since there is only one simulation time step. In the case of multiple time steps, the concentration on the diffusion front is time dependent and might underrun a chosen constant threshold. This is illustrated in Fig.8.4. With a solver that is stable enough not to produce artificial negative concentration values the threshold can be chosen to be close enough to zero not to let that happen. Otherwise the subzero regions discussed before in section 8.2 present a problem. Even for the more stable SG2 simulation results,

8.3. The TOA Map

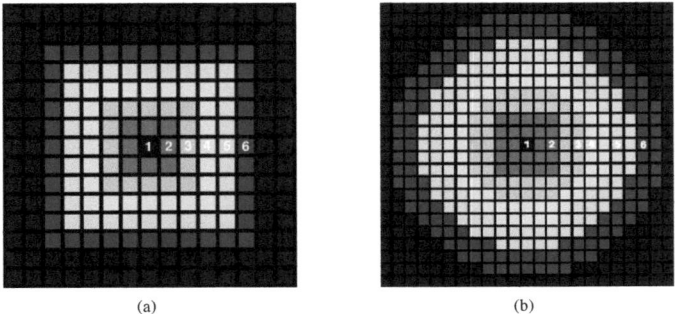

Figure 8.3.: *A comparison of the TOAs of the fast marching method (a) and the DSBT method (b). The DSBT method covers more data points in one time step. The steps in the TOA are wider than in the one created by the fast-marching technique.*

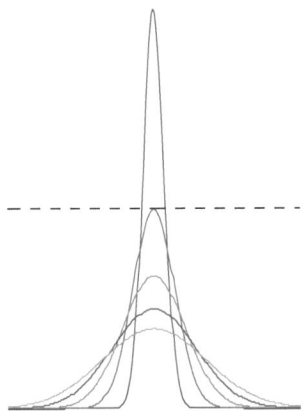

Figure 8.4.: *The concentration (colored curves) may underrun a constant threshold (stipled line) if several time steps are evaluated.*

8. Diffusion Simulation Based Tracking

classification with a fixed threshold close to zero is not advisable because the distance between the diffusion fronts of two successive simulation steps varies considerably. The gap to the previous front gets narrower for each time step. I therefore evaluated other time step dependent concentration thresholds TH for the determination of the diffusion front.

$TH = max_c(t) * k$: $max_c(t)$ is the maximal concentration value encountered in the simulation step t. k is a constant that describes the position of the concentration threshold in relation to $max_c(t)$. This method produces an expansion covering (almost) the whole evaluated volume, depending on the chosen k (see Fig.8.5(a) and 8.5(d)). For small k few time steps are enough to cover the whole volume. The flooded region, in this case, is large for each time step, especially so for the first time step. Even if the k is adjusted, so that the flooded regions are in general smaller, the region for the first step remains large in comparison.

$TH = max_c(t) k^{t/const}$: This method results for $const = 100$ in an expansion covering (almost) the whole evaluated volume. There is still some variance in the breadth of the different TOA fronts (see Fig.8.5(b) and 8.5(e)).

$TH = max_c(t) * k^{t/t_{max}}$: This function will return a regular expansion but it will not cover the whole volume in the same time the previous functions do (see Fig.8.5(c) and 8.5(f)).

In Fig.8.3 the thresholding of the concentration peak is illustrated in the lower row for the first four simulation time steps on a vertical cut through a 2D concentration peak. The threshold of the peak in time t is plotted as stippled line in the same color as the concentration peak in time t. In the upper row the resulting TOA map for a maximum of 20 time steps is shown. The coloring in both plots in each column is the same for the individual time steps. The regions covered by a single diffusion step have individual widths as can be seen in Fig.8.5. This is easily observable in the top views given in Fig.8.5(a)-8.5(c).

To have even more controll over the distance between adjacent fronts, a histogram based classification was evaluated. A concentration histogram for a given time step is divided into equally sized concentration intervals (see Fig.8.6). Until a predefined minimal number of points is reached, the interval corresponding to the next largest concentration is flooded. This method guarantees a minimal number of flooded points per time step. Only data points that were not flooded previously are considered on building the histogram to guarantee that additional points are flooded in each time step. This histogram based method proved useful for the evaluation of the FEMLAB simulations since the concentration threshold for these results needed to be very high to avoid problems with value dips caused by non-monotone concentration decrease. For the more stable results gained from SG2 the threshold $TH = max_c(t) * (1 - 99.9\%)^{t/10}$ returns well spaced diffusion fronts with a relative small region covered in the first time step and is less computational intensive than the histogram based classification.

8.3. The TOA Map

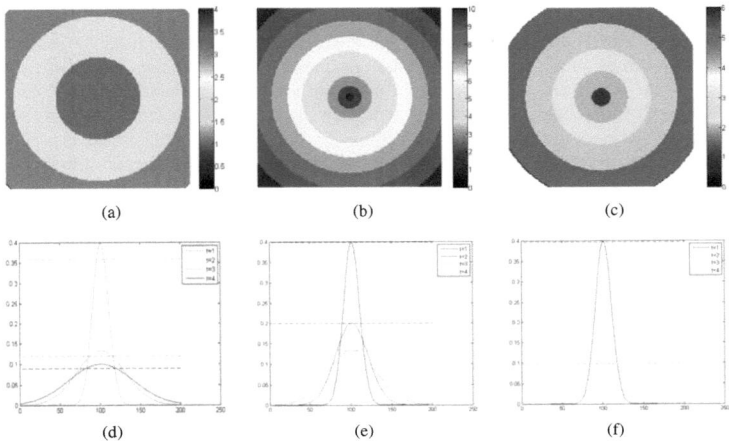

Figure 8.5.: *The detection of the diffusion fronts illustrated on the example of isotropic diffusion in 2D. The main difference between the methods is the size of the flooded region for the individual time steps.*

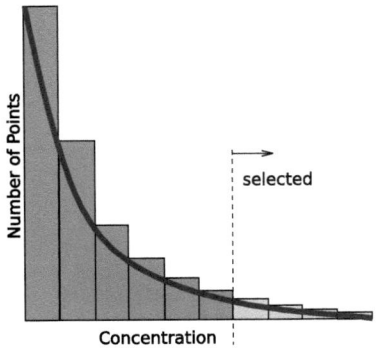

Figure 8.6.: *The method of histogram classification is illustrated here. The classification threshold is chosen to guarantee a predefined minimal number of points to be flooded in each time step.*

8.4. The Gradient Descend

In the next step of the algorithm the actual tract reconstruction takes place. A tract is reconstructed by following a gradient, starting from a point on the outermost diffusion front in the TOA map, and descending from there toward the simulation origin which corresponds to the center of the initial peak (see Fig.8.7). The backtracking character of this reconstruction handles fiber branching conveniently. The arms of the branches reunite automatically on the way back to the origin. The maximal amount of branches that is admissible in a reconstruction is predefined by the user. The number of allowed branches determines the required computation time.

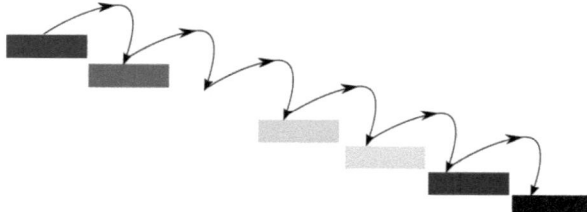

Figure 8.7.: *The gradient descend reconstructs a tract from the outermost front (dark red) in the TOA map toward the simulation origin (dark blue). The different time stamps in the TOA map are illustrated as colored bars.*

A first idea for the computation of the gradients was to compute them directly on the TOA map entries. The tract is then reconstructed by following the negative gradient direction toward the simulation origin. When the distance between two adjacent fronts is small enough, as for example in the fast-marching TOA maps (see Fig.8.3), this gradient can be computed by central differences of the map entries. In the case of TOA map based DSBT this is generally not the case.

An other idea is to connect the points on adjacent fronts with straight lines, in analogy to the DSBT in [51]. This will result in a very large number of possible tracts because all points in the radius given by the smoothing conditions might give a valid connection, as illustrated in Fig.8.8. The gradient descend starts in a point on the outermost front (red star). All straight connections with the next diffusion front, which do not violate the smoothness criteria, need to be evaluated (red triangle). In the next step, all possible connections to the next inner diffusion front need to be investigated for all points on the diffusion front inside the triangle, defined by the smoothness conditions (green stars) and so on until the diffusion seed is reached. Of all these possible tracts, the ones that connect a point on the outermost diffusion front with the simulation seed, need to be evaluated. The number of possible tracts ($T_{possible}$) increases at most exponentially with the number of time stamps (t_{max}) in the TOA map ($T_{possible} = N^{t_{max}}$, with N the number of connections possible in the given smoothness restrictions). This number is reduced

8.4. The Gradient Descend

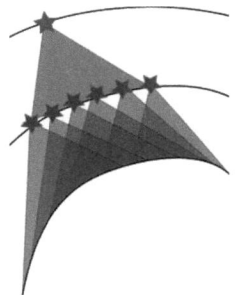

Figure 8.8.: *The increase in possible tracts for each simulation time step is illustrated here.*

due to the decrease in the surface corresponding to the next smaller time stamp in the TOA but still it remains large. Not only does the large number of possible connections between two adjacent diffusion fronts present a problem for the individual connections. Bridging between diffusion fronts causes the tracking results to encompass more unlikely connections that would have terminated in between the diffusion fronts. Actual pathways might also be excluded because detailed curving between the diffusion fronts is ignored, causing the reconstruction to violate the smoothness criteria. All in all, the reliability of the tracking results is considerably reduced by such a straight connection in between diffusion fronts that are several voxels apart.

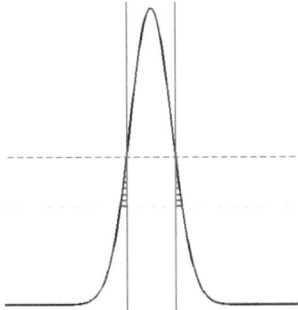

Figure 8.9.: *The concentration values of all points flooded the first time in a time step (blue striped region, between stippled lines) is used to compute the concentration values. The region between the red lines was previously flooded and is therefore not considered in this step.*

8. Diffusion Simulation Based Tracking

The question of interpolation on the TOA map needs to be addressed to get better determined pathways between two adjacent diffusion fronts. The interpolation on the sparse grid of diffusion front points is not trivial and requires additional computations to generate the gradients on the TOA map time stamps. An alternative is the use of concentration gradients computed from simulation results (see Fig.8.9). The concentration values from the simulation step that first reaches a point is stored to compute the concentration gradient later on with simple direct differences. This easy generation method reduces the required amount of computations. The gradient in the simulation seed is set to zero. The concentration gradient was preferred for this DSBT method because of its easy and fast computability.

8.5. Problems With The Single Simulation Approach

Artifacts will occur if only one simulation is used to propagate the front over the whole data set. There are two very prominent artifacts that prevent DSBT from expanding over a whole data set in one go.

Firstly, the fact that the diffusivity outside the fiber tracts is nonzero because of noise or anatomy causes bleeding of the diffusion fronts outside the actual tracts. The problems this bleeding may cause are illustrated on the example of two synthetic fiber pathways. In simple cases, as illustrated in Fig.8.10, the bleeding artifacts can be filtered by thresholding the anisotropy similar to the tract termination criterion presented in section 7.1.1.1. The simulation results are only considered in voxels with high anisotropy (see Fig.8.10(b)). More complicated tract structures lead to more problematic bleeding

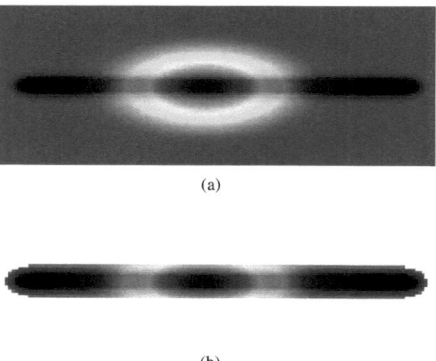

(a)

(b)

Figure 8.10.: *The simulation and therefore the TOA map will bleed into the background if diffusivity outside of the fiber is not ideally zero (a). The background can be filtered by thresholding the anisotropy, as shown in (b).*

8.5. Problems With The Single Simulation Approach

artifacts. This is illustrated on the example of a spiral fiber in Fig.8.11. The diffusion is following the tract nicely in the beginning but because of bleeding throughout the background the inner part of the spiral is reached by the bleeding diffusion front before the diffusion front that follows the spiral path reaches it. Filtering the resulting fronts with an FA threshold will not greatly improve the results because faulty TOA entries will remain on the tract. The faulty TOA entries will cause faulty gradients which will not follow the path of the fiber that is to be reconstructed but the course of the bleeding. The reconstruction will fail in these faulty TOA regions. Since the transition between gradients following the fiber and the ones following the bleeding direction are in general non-smooth, the tract reconstruction will be terminated where true and faulty TOA entries meet.

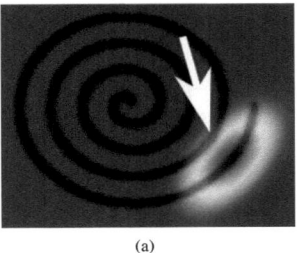
(a)

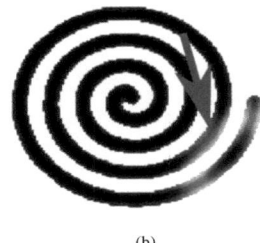
(b)

Figure 8.11.: *The simulated diffusion in (a) is bleeding into the background and from there again into the spiral. (b) shows that the bleeding in the background can be masked by anisotropy thresholding but on reentering the tract it will cause problems for the tracking algorithm. The region where the diffusion is entering the inner winding of the spiral through the background is indicated with an arrow in each image.*

Anisotropy thresholding could in theory also be applied during the simulation process or as a preprocessing step preventing 'background bleeding' completely. In the preprocessing the tensor entries of a tensor in a voxel with low anisotropy might be set to zero. The so applied anisotropy threshold might affect the simulation results since the complete tensor information in the evaluated neighborhood is considered during the simulation process. It needs to be evaluated how grave the difference in the simulation results is and whether the early application of the anisotropy threshold shows advantages over the thresholding used in the here presented implementation.

Secondly, the initial concentration needs to be increased to be able to cover the whole data set with one simulation. For a dirac initialization this will increase the distance between the concentration value in the ROI and the background concentration of zero. This will increase the artifacts, caused by the non-continuous dirac-like initialization. To gain a more stable simulation result the initialization needs to have smoother transitions to the background causing the previously discussed artificial expansion of the user defined ROI (see Fig.8.1). This results in a gap between the reconstructed tract and the user defined

8. Diffusion Simulation Based Tracking

ROI that needs to be bridged. Tracking is usually performed in more than one direction starting in the ROI. Bridging the gap, which results from widening of the peak, can cause non-smooth connections between the tract pieces. The phenomenon is illustrated in Fig.8.12.

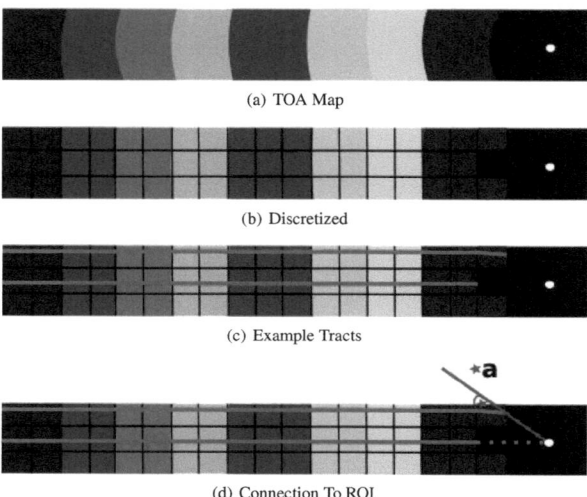

Figure 8.12.: *An illustration of the straight line bridging of the gap between the boundary of the initial peak (dark blue on the right) and the original ROI (white dot). (a) shows the TOA map of a simple fiber example. This map is discretized to the data grid in (b). In (c) two exemplary reconstructed tracts are plotted in gray over the TOA map. In (d) the trackts are connected to the original ROI with a straight line.*

Fig.8.12(a) shows a TOA map which is the basis of the tract reconstruction. The background is masked by anisotropy filtering. No tracking is possible here therefore no TOA values are computed in the background. The individual time steps are marked with individual colors. The center of each expanding front is the original seed (white point). The fronts are therefore less curved the further they are away from this seed. Due to discretization the fronts run in parallel to each other (orthogonal to the axis of the fiber) from the second times step onwards. The discretization eliminates low curvature of the individual fronts. In Fig.8.12(c) two exemplary tracts are shown overlayed on the TOA map. The tracts run smoothly until they reach the outer boundary of the initial peak (dark blue region on the right). The gap between the boundary of the initial peak could be bridged with a straight line as illustrated in Fig.8.12(d) by the dotted extensions of the fibers. For the tract that runs in the center of the fiber the straight connection to the original ROI is a direct extension of the tract and no smoothness criteria are violated. This straight connection with the original ROI is not necessarily smooth as illustrated on the second fiber in Fig.8.12(d). An angle a exists between the reconstructed tract and the straight line connecting the tract to the original ROI. If this angle a is to large (larger than the smoothness criteria permit) the reconstruction cannot be smoothly connected to the original ROI by a straight line. This gap could in theory be bridged with the concentration gradient of the initial peak but this connection will not depend on the underlying anatomy because the peak has not yet started to diffuse. The concentration gradient can therefore not establish reliable connections with the user defined ROI.

8.6. Successive Simulations

To overcome the problems of the single simulation approach, successive simulations are performed on subgrids which cover a small region in the data set. The definition of a

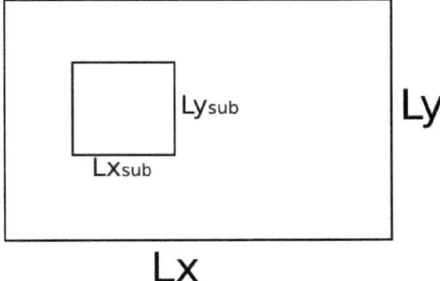

Figure 8.13.: *The subgrid is a small region in the data volume.*

subgrid is illustrated in Fig.8.13 in 2D. Lx is the length of the data grid in X-direction ($Lx = \#x \Delta x$ with $\#x$ the number of voxels and Δx the size of the voxels in x direction). Lx_{sub} is the length of the subgrid, which is smaller than the data grid ($Lx_{sub} = \alpha Lx$ with $\alpha \leq 1$). Ly and Ly_{sub} are defined in the same way. Throughout the tract reconstruction the size of the subgrid is fixed for all simulations.

The subregions need not have the same voxel resolution as the original data set but can be regridded to any resolution. Therefore, α can be chosen arbitrarily. As mentioned before in the description of the SG2 simulation solver in section 8.2.2, the accuracy of the simulation results increases with an increase in subgrid resolution that is the number of voxels in the subgrid $\#x_{sub}$ in each dimension because the resulting reduction in the individual subvoxel volume corresponds to a reduction in the control volume size. The subgrid resolution $\#x_{sub}$ is the same for all subgrids in a tract reconstruction.

In the tract reconstruction the simulation is now evaluated on overlapping subgrids. The first subgrid is constructed to have the centroid of the user defined ROI voxel as

8. Diffusion Simulation Based Tracking

center. On this subgrid, all steps of the reconstruction are performed (section 8.2-8.4). The end points of the tract pieces that were reconstructed in this region are used as future simulation seeds. For each of these future simulation seeds a new subregion with a simulation seed as centroid is defined. On this new subgrid all steps of DSBT are also evaluated. The corresponding tract piece end points are again considered as future seeds. In this fashion successive simulations are performed along the fiber that is to be reconstructed until DSBT has evaluated all future simulation seeds.

The tract pieces are later on concatenated to form the whole fiber tract reconstructions. The successive evaluation is illustrated in Fig.8.14. The reconstruction starts at the leftmost black dot which depicts the original ROI. The red line represents the reconstructed tract. It consists of individual pieces that are connected at the black dots which represent the simulation seeds. The simulation results are represented in this illustration as black lines that give the outermost diffusion front. Points that would cause the tract to turn back toward the last simulation seed are excluded from the evaluation, because the smoothness criteria do not allow sharp turns in the tracts. The plane that divides the simulation results into points that are ignored (stippled line in the second simulation result) and points that need further processing (black line), is depicted by a dotted black line. The arrows that are attached to this line indicate the side of the plane that contains the points that are to be further processed. The simulations can have multiple extrema as illustrated on the right of Fig.8.14. Multiple extrema will cause branching in the tract.

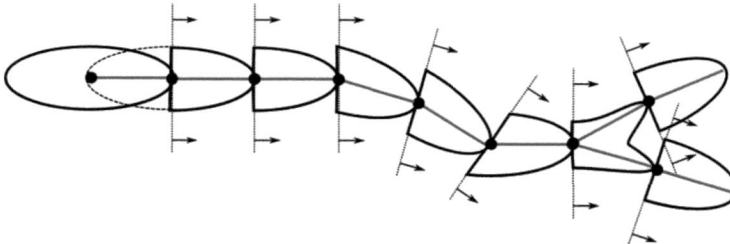

Figure 8.14.: *This graphic illustrates the successive evaluation of the diffusion simulation on small subregions. The simulation results are depicted as black lines that represent the outermost diffusion front. The black dot marks the simulation origin. The red line stands for the reconstructed tract piece. From the second simulation onward, the number of points, that can be part of a valid tract, are reduced because of the smoothness criteria. The reduction of the points is illustrated with the dotted black cutting plane. The arrows attached to this plane indicate, which part of the diffusion front will be considered in the evaluation.*

To avoid that the boundary condition (concentration is zero on the boundary; see section 8.2.2) affects the simulation results that are used for further processing in the reconstruction a boundary of $\#b$ voxel is chosen to surround the subgrid that is used in the

8.6. Successive Simulations

tracking $\#x_{use}$ as illustrated in Fig.8.15. The subgrid voxel (also known as subvoxel) resolution in each dimension is, therefore, $\#x_{sub} = \#x_{use} + 2\#b$.

For the SG2 sovlver $\#b = 6$ was chosen. This is more than enough since this solver is very accurate and the boundary only affects the voxels next to the boundary in a dramatic way. With the SG2 solver the effect of the boundary condition is less dramatic than the one in the FEMLAB solver, which requires a border of at least 10 subvoxel in each direction.

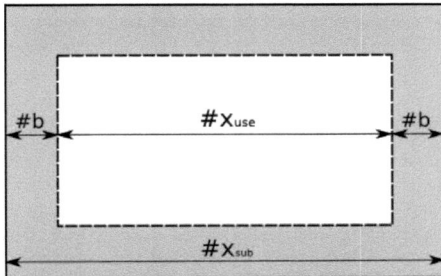

Figure 8.15.: *To avoid effects of the boundary condition a border is introduced to the subgrid.*

8.6.1. Known Problems

In the next paragraphs I want to discuss some known problems of the successive evaluation of subgrids and their solutions. The problems can usually be solved by tuning the parameters of the tracking algorithm.

8.6.1.1. Branching in the First Simulation

To controll the computation time the maximal number of branches in each subgrid evaluation is fixed for the reconstruction. Only the first few points, in a list sorted according to their distance to the seed in descending order, are considered as future simulation seeds. Points with the same distance from the seed that exceed the permitted number of branching are ignored.

If the amount of branching is restricted to, for example, two branches it is highly probable that two points that are close to each other on the diffusion front are chosen as seeds for further simulations. This is not a problem for the reconstruction in later subgrid evaluations but for the initial subgrid this could lead (in the case of an ellipsoid diffusion profile) to a dominance of one of the directions corresponding to the principal diffusion orientation over the other since the distance from the original seed points is usually the same for both directions and a small region surrounding the extrema. The

8. Diffusion Simulation Based Tracking

number of allowed branches was, therefore, increased for the first simulation to increase the probability that all major diffusion directions are considered.

The selection of future seed points is in part chance because only a fixed number of points is chosen depending only on their distance from the simulation seed, not their actual position. This behavior could be improved if further criteria are used to select the future seed points. For example, a minimal distance between the points could be enforced or a local minimum in the surface of the outermost diffusion front could be used to separate two future seed points. A weighting of the distance with FA value in the possible future seed could also be used, so that tract pieces ending in more anisotropic regions are preferred. This should keep the tract closer to the more anisotropic center of the fiber.

8.6.1.2. Falsely Isotropic Diffusion Simulation

The simulation parameters (duration of a single simulation step and number of these steps) have to be tuned with care. A small number of short simulation steps may result in falsely isotropic TOA maps if the anisotropy is not very strong, since a certain amount of change in the position of the simulated diffusion is needed take effect on the extracted diffusion front that is stored in the discrete TOA map. If the change in a simulation time step to small (less than a voxel) this change will not register in the TOA map.

DSBT can (to some extend) still reconstruct some fibers on isotropic TOA maps and will not terminate straight away as other tracking algorithms do if their parameters are chosen inadequately. The FA value of the measured diffusion tensors do not determine the falsely isotropic TOA and therefore are not necessarily low. This is the reason why no tract termination criterion is violated in the beginning of the reconstruction and the reconstruction is not aborted. The reconstruction starts in the first simulation by selecting

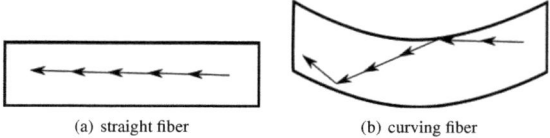

(a) straight fiber   (b) curving fiber

Figure 8.16.: *When the simulated diffusion is isotropic, the fiber will be reconstructed as straight line until a boundary is reached. The effect is most prominent in curving fibers (b).*

the points on the isotropic diffusion front by chance because all points have the same distance to the seed point. From the so selected points the tracking will continue in a straight line until the border of the fiber is reached (as illustrated in Fig.8.16(b)). Here, the reconstruction will change direction and follow another straight line until it meets another fiber boundary or it terminates because smoothness criteria are violated. The smoothness criteria that are applied to the tracts prefer straight reconstructions and therefore will enforce, if possible, the selection of points on a straight path as future seeds. Especially in straight fibers (see Fig.8.16(a)) it is almost impossible to determine if the simulated diffusion was isotropic from the reconstructed tracts. Even in curving tracts it is in actual reconstructions not always obvious. To avoid falsely isotropic simulation results the simulation time and the number of simulation steps need to be chosen appropriately. A good choice is a minimum of 20 simulation steps with a simulation time of 0.001s which covers an isotropic subgrid corresponding to $15 \times 15 \times 1.6$ data voxels in the synthetic datasets evaluated in the results section 8.9.

8.7. Tracking Acceleration

The computation time for the complete reconstruction grows exponentially with the increase in simulation seeds, i.e. branches, for this tracking algorithm. To reduce computation time, the number of simulation seeds needs to be minimal. A first step in this direction allows only a low number of branches for the tract reconstruction. This does reduce the total computation time dramatically but even with a low number of branching (allowed branches = 2), the total computation time is dependent on the tract length and can be several days, with a simulation time of approximately 43s on a subgrid (see section 8.6 for more on subgrids) that covers 15 x 15 x 1.6 voxels in a regridded resolution of 65 x 65 x 65. The tracking time on the so computed simulation results is approximately 0.117s.

The isotropic regridding of the subgrid results in a finer resuolution in Z-direction in comparison with the X- and Y-direction. In the reconstruction of 3D geometries this might bias the tracking results. For the here presented theoretical evaluation it has no effect.

All evaluations were performed on a PC with on an Intel Quad-Core Xeon E5320 processor with 1.86GHz and 4GB RAM. Only one processor was used for each evaluation, parallel processing could therefore also provide further acceleration of the algorithm.

To accelerate the evaluation on a single processor more termination criteria were developed, which will be discussed in the following. It is important to note that the aim of these criteria is the reduction of computation time, not the elimination of anatomically improbable tracts. When the computation time is irrelevant, more accurate results might be achievable without the following criteria.

8.7.1. Subgrid Resolution

The speed of the simulation is dependent on the resolution of the subgrid, that is the number of subgrid voxels. The actual resolution of the subgrid in the data dimension is assumed to be constant (10% of the datagrid dimension). Subgrid resolution here means the number of subvoxels in each dimension. A simulation time step of 0.001s and and 20 successive simulation steps are used in this evaluation. For an isotropic subgrid resolution of 65 a complete simulation takes approximately 25s. For an isotropic subgrid resolution of 45 it takes approximately 12s and for a subgrid resolution of 33 approximately 5s. The time that is required for the tract reconstruction on the simulation results

8. Diffusion Simulation Based Tracking

is always considerably less than 1s. It is approximately 0.1s for an isotropic subgrid resolution of 65, 0.03s for a resolution of 45 and 0.005 for a resolution of 33. The number of subvoxels will determine the stepsize in the gradient descend which corresponds to one subvoxel length. The higher the subvoxel resolution, the smaller the steps. The time needed for the complete evaluation naturally increases with the number of subvoxels since this increases the number of points to be processed. One has to find a good trade off between subvoxel resolution and reconstruction time. Usually an isotropic subgrid resolution between 33 or 45 is sufficient. The number of subvoxels should be odd and to allow the maximal use of multigrids it should ideally be $2^c + 1$ (with c a constant).

The size and resolution of the evaluated subgrid needs to be chosen to match the other simulation parameters. If it is too small or the resolution is too low, most of the simulated diffusion fronts will be discarded since only those fronts are considered that lie completely inside the evaluated subgrid (without considering the subgrid border) to avoid influence of the border conditions and to be able to consider the complete shape of the front. The influence of the subgrid resolution on the tracking results is also discussed in section 8.9.1.2.

8.7.2. The Similarity Tract Termination Criterion

This tract termination criterion is used to reduce the number of similar tracts in the reconstruction. If two tracts are considered similar they are merged so that only one tract is further propagated.

If two tract pieces end in the same data grid voxel they are tested for similarity. To determine the similarity the last few steps in both tract reconstructions are compared. If the distance between the tracts in these few steps is below a given threshold they are considered similar. In this case the tracts will be merged in this point and continue along the same path. The tracking needs not be further propagated for both tract pieces simultaneously because they will follow (approximately) the same path. The tracking is continued on the first tract piece reaching the point of merger. The reconstruction is aborted at the first simulation seed after the tracts overlap for tracts which will reach the point of merger at a later time in the reconstruction.

The abortion of similar tracts will influence the results because similar tracts are not necessarily completely equal from the point of merger onward. Detailed tract variations are lost because one of the tracts is aborted, if two similar tracts are merged. My investigations did show that this kind of tract reduction does not affect the reconstruction severely on the evaluated synthetic data sets as is shown later on in section 8.9.1.1. DSBT with the similarity tract termination does still reconstruct the fibers completely but not with as many individual tracts.

The merging of tracts is illustrated in Fig.8.17 where two tracts merge because the distance d is smaller than a chosen threshold C_s. The tract on top is aborted after the merger, the lower one continues. The simulation seeds are again given by black dots (similar to Fig.8.14) and the reconstructed tract pieces are given by red lines. The direction of the successive reconstruction is indicated by small black arrows on dotted lines that determine which parts of the simulation results are to be considered for the reconstruction.

8.7. Tracking Acceleration

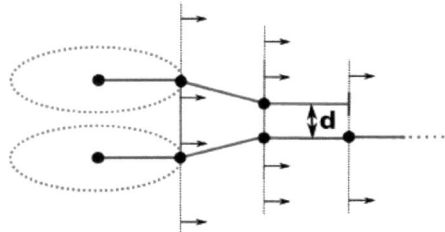

Figure 8.17.: *Merger of the path of two tracts that are similar ($d < C_s$).*

This is implemented with a map containing all processed simulation endpoints and the corresponding reconstruction keys, which identify the reconstructed tract piece. When a reconstruction of a tract piece is finished, the endpoints that are to be added to the queue of simulation seeds are compared to this map. If there is an entry, the reconstructions might be similar. The endpoint of the similar tract is not added to the queue awaiting further processing and the tract is classified as aborted. The classification is also described in Alg.:1. Here tract [] is an array containing the points of the current tract piece.

Algorithm 1 Similarity (tract, previouslyReconstructedTracts)

1: endVoxel = tract[end]
2: reference = previouslyReconstructedTracts[endVoxel]
3: **if** reference is empty **then**
4:     **return false**
5: **else**
6:     **for** $i = 0$ to 2 **do**
7:         p1 = tract[i]
8:         p2 = reference[i]
9:         **if** $|p1, p2| \geq C_s$ **then**
10:             **return false**
11: **return true**

The array reference [] contains a tract the was previously reconstructed and ends in the same data voxel. The map previouslyReconstructedTracts [] contains all reconstructed tract pieces. The tract pieces can be accessed by the voxel they end in (endVoxel) which is the identifying key in this map. If no previous reconstruction ends in the same voxel as the current one reference will be empty. In line 6 to 10 of Alg.:1 the last three reconstruction steps on both tract pieces are compared. In line 9 |p1, p2| stands for the distance between the coordinate vectors of p1 on the current tract and p2 on the previously reconstructed tract. If Alg.:1 returns TRUE the reconstruction continues for both tract pieces. Otherwise the reconstruction for the current tract piece is aborted because it is merged with the previously reconstructed tract piece.

8. Diffusion Simulation Based Tracking

The criterion was evaluated on a synthetic branching fiber from the PISTE data sets [25]. More information on the data set is given in the results section 8.9. For $C_s = 1e^{-4}$ the number of aborted tracts is approximately three percent of the total number of reconstructed tracts. The number of abortions increases to approximately ten percent for $C_s = 0.1$. The total computation time for the reconstruction is still several days with an isotropic subgrid resolution of 33. The threshold was further increased to $C_s = 1$, which led to an abortion rate of approximately 90 percent and a computation time of 8.5 hours. This also drastically reduces the number of tracts. I chose $C_s = 0.5$ for the evaluation because this value presents a good trade-off between the number of reconstructed tracts and speed. The effect of the similarity threshold on the tracking results is also discussed in section 8.9.1.1.

8.7.3. Global Smoothness Tract Termination

A global smoothness criterion was introduced to accelerate DSBT on the synthetic data sets. This criterion is used to eliminate tracts with strong curving by thresholding the angle between the averaged tract piece directions (see Fig.8.18). This criterion will reduce the number of tracts, thereby reducing the computation time.

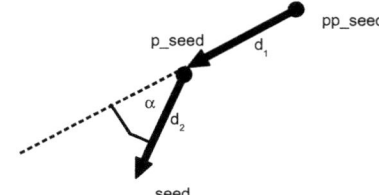

Figure 8.18.: *The global smoothness depends on the angle α between the average tract directions d_i. The first tract reconstructs a path between pp_seed and p_seed. The second one starts in p_seed and ends in seed.*

The average tract direction vector d_i ($i \in 1, 2$) is computed by subtracting the coordinate vectors of the end point and origin of a tract piece. The average tract direction vector is normalized to a length of one ($\overline{d_i} = d_i/|d_i|$). The dot product of the average normalized tract direction vectors of two adjoining tract pieces is related to the angle α separating them (8.8).

$$cos(\alpha) = \overline{d_1}.\overline{d_2} \qquad (8.8)$$

To guarantee a maximal angle between two tract pieces, the tracts are terminated if $cos(\alpha) > TH$. To allow all kinds of curving tracts, the threshold TH should equal zero. To allow no curving, it should be one. Tract pieces that do not satisfy this global smoothness condition are discarded.

This criterion does not reduce the number of tracts as dramatically as the similarity threshold. The improvement of the computation time, therefore, is relatively small. The global restriction of curving might prevent the reconstruction of the strong curving fiber pathways. This restrictive parameter therefore needs to be carefully tuned. The expected advantage of the restriction needs to outweigh the effect on the tracking. In practice this criterion is not very effective. Only few tracts are terminated even if the threshold is high (TH = 0.9 corresponds to a maximal angle of 25.8 degrees). The gain does not justify the additional computation time required to apply this criterion. It was therefore rejected.

A variation of this criterion might be usable to restrict branching in regions of crossing with a relatively small angle between the crossing fibers. In such cases the tracking will follow all possible directions from the region of crossing, causing the reconstructed tract to branch and generate false positive connections. An example can be seen in section 8.9.3. The criterion would need to use the mean direction over several simulations, rendering the tract less flexible. The advantage of such a restrictive criterion needs to be carefully investigated in the future.

8.7.4. Look-Up-Table

The reconstruction with DSBT is compared to the SLT method very time consuming. To accelerate the actual tract reconstruction, the simulation results for all possible subgrids (one for each voxel in the data set) can be computed in a preprocessing step. This reduces repeated computations of simulations originating in the same voxel. This is especially important for extensive evaluations with multiple ROIs on a single data set. The precomputed subgrid results are stored in a look-up-table (LUT). The ideal LUT for DSBT would contain the complete simulation results for overlapping subregions (similar to the ones used in the successive evaluation described in section 8.5), one corresponding to each voxel in the data set, thereby evading restriction of the tracking algorithms by restricting the data. This, however, leads to extensive usage of hard disc storage space (a little over 30 GB for a 192x192 pixel slice with subregions containing 10^3 data grid voxels (subgrid voxel size = data grid voxel size) and evaluated for 20 simulation steps), rendering the ideal LUT unsuitable for the goal of efficient fiber tracking on commonly available computers. To reduce the amount of storage needed, a TOA map is computed from the simulation results and stored for each subgrid instead of the original simulation results (TOA-LUT). The whole simulation result for a subgrid with an isotropic subgrid resolution of 10 and 20 time steps consists of 20.000 concentration values (type double) plus 20.000 time values (type float), whereas the TOA map only contains 1.000 time values (type float). Additional gradients contain 3.000 values (type float). Using a TOA-LUT with additional gradients therefore saves approximately 93 percent of the storage needed per subgrid.

The TOA map in a subgrid with low diffusion contribution in the simulation seed (centroid) is not important for the reconstruction. Its contribution to the reconstruction (if there is one) is covered in the neighboring subgrids with stronger diffusion profiles that also contain this voxel with low diffusion contribution. The computation time for an entry corresponding to a subgrid with low diffusion contribution, evaluated for second order diffusion tensor data in the TOA-LUT, is roughly 24 seconds in Matlab/Femlab and approximately 2 seconds in SG2.

8. Diffusion Simulation Based Tracking

To make the LUT computation even more efficient means to identify these low diffusion contribution subgrids to avoid computation of superfluous entries need to be defined. For the identification of low diffusivity subgrids, the diffusion tensor corresponding to the simulation seed (centroid) of each subgrid needs to be classified according to the corresponding diffusion profile. The simulation seed has a large influence on the diffusion inside a subgrid because this is where the initial concentration peak is defined for the simulation (see section 8.2). The voxels surrounding the simulation seed in the subgrid have their own corresponding LUT entries, for which they are the centroid, and therefore need not be considered in the classification of the current subgrid.

There are several choices for the classification parameter. One possibility for the classification of diffusion tensors is the mean diffusivity (see (4.10)). Another way to classify the diffusion in this context is the fractional anisotropy (see (4.12)). In fiber tracking isotropic regions have low fractional anisotropy and are of no interest. In the tracking process a fractional anisotropy threshold is used as termination criterion for reconstructed tracts. When this parameter is set in the LUT, it should be selected sufficiently low because it can not be lowered later on without recomputation of the LUT. The anisotropy threshold for the elimination of surplus LUT entries cannot exceed the threshold used for tracking.

The filtered LUT will be irregular, meaning that not every voxel in the data set has a corresponding LUT entry. This irregularity has to be considered when tracking is performed on the LUT data. For the tracking process only 'reachable' LUT-entries are important. An entry is reachable if at least one of its 26 possible neighbors on the 3D data grid exists. The application of the previously discussed filtering criteria make it possible that LUT-entries have no neighbors. These isolated subgrids can be eliminated prior to LUT generation with a simple preprocessing step. The filter criterion is a threshold for the a scalar diffusion index used to eliminate surplus LUT entries. This index can be easily computed for the whole data set. If for a given voxel all 26 neighbors have index values below this threshold, the voxel is isolated. The isolated voxels are disregarded in the LUT.

The LUT contains only entries for non-isolated subgrids with high diffusion index values. This will save computation time by reducing the number of unnecessary simulations as well as storage space. The computations for the LUT are still time consuming and therefore only advisable for datasets requiring more extensive connectivity investigations that evaluate the tracking algorithm in several ROIs.

8.7.5. Propagator Approach

Another possibility to accelerate the tracking replaces the computationally costly simulation step with a simpler evaluation of the propagator. The propagator can be used as a crude approximation of the diffusion front corresponding to a short simulation step. For the standard second order tensor, the propagator is an ellipsoid. This ellipse has only one dominant orientation when it is cigar shaped and an infinite number of equally dominant directions in any other case (disc or sphere). The algorithm would work similarly to the SLT method and also have the same problems (see also sections 7.1.1.2 and 8.9). The advantage of handling, for example, crossing fibers cannot be resolved by this kind of propagator approach since the propagators in the region of crossing do (in general) not correspond to the direction of the fiber tracts. An example is given in Fig.8.26, where the orientation of the ellipsoids is the average of the two orientations of the ellipsoids that actually correspond to the fiber tracts. The fibers that are reconstructed from the propagator can only follow this false orientation. The distortion can be reduced for small regions of crossing by interpolation of the propagators. The distorted orientation can be somewhat corrected by the interpolation. In the case of orthogonal crossing the propagator can become disc-shaped. In this case it would be impossible to determine a dominant direction from the propagator. Two points on the surface of the propagator would be chosen by chance. I rejected the idea of a second order tensor propagator based DSBT variation because all the advantages this method has over SLT, especially the handling of crossing and curving tracts (see section 8.9 for a comparison of the reconstruction results), would be lost.

Propagators for more advanced diffusion representations might overcome these problems. The advantage of such a propagator approach over a simulation based reconstruction needs to be investiagted.

8.8. Implementation

The implementation follows the three steps of the DSBT algorithm that were presented in section 8.2-8.4. Each step is implemented in its own class. An overview over the classes is given in Fig.8.19. The individual steps are coordinated and information is passed on in the main DSBT method. A more detailed description is given in the flow chart 8.20. Here, the class structure is color coded. This makes it easier to determine, which step is performed by which module of the implementation and where the modules interact. This chart also gives a short overview over the individual steps of the algorithm that were discussed in more detail in the previous sections.

8. Diffusion Simulation Based Tracking

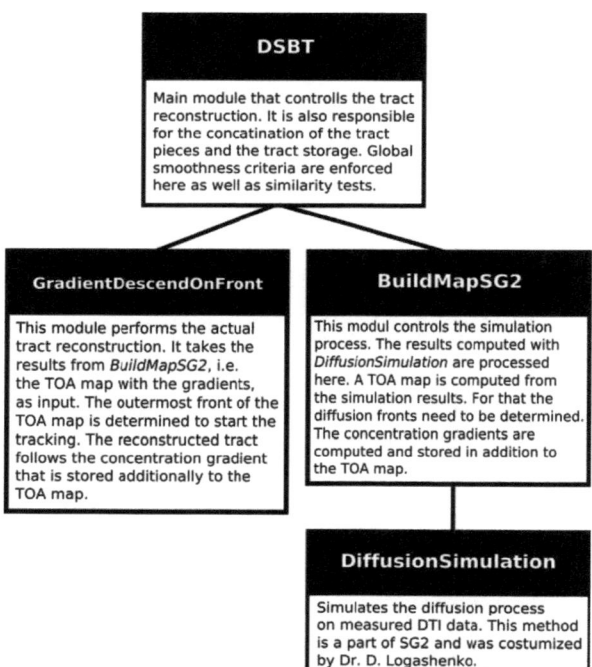

Figure 8.19.: *An overview over the class structure of the implementation.*

8.9. Tracking Results

The DSBT algorithm introduced here was evaluated on synthetic DTI data for validation purposes. The Phantom Images for Simulating Tractography Errors (PISTE) proposed and published by Deoni and Jones [25] were used because they cover a large range of fiber tracts which may cause problems for commonly used reconstruction methods. The tracts were generated by simulating a DTI measurement with 30 DWI and 4 unweighted images. A ForcePairs GES with 30 directions was used. The TE in the simulated measurements was 90ms. A b-factor of 1000s/mm^2 was chosen. The T_2 time on the tract is 65ms and 95ms in the background. The data grid for the here evaluated data sets has a size of $150 \times 150 \times 16$ voxels with isotropic voxel side length. For the diffusion simulation of DSBT the preprocessed tensors were used as input. Some of the reconstructed geometries are presented in the following. To demonstrate the big advantages that DSBT

8.9. Tracking Results

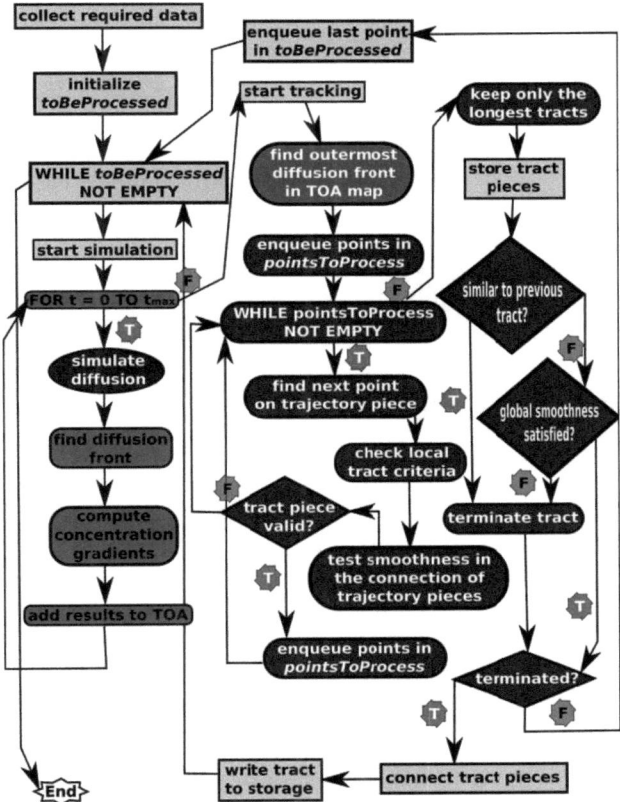

Figure 8.20.: *A flow chart of the algorithm. The steps are color and shape coded, according to the class they belong to: green - rectangular corresponds to the main DSBT method; red - round rectangles correspond to BuildMapSG2; dark red - oval, corresponds to the SG2 simulation and blue - stretched circle corresponds to GradientDescendOnFront. The small red signs (F) mark the path taken when the loop condition or the condition in the corresponding diamond is false, the green signs (T) mark paths for true conditions.*

8. Diffusion Simulation Based Tracking

has over commonly used tracking methods and also to illustrate the problems of the individual fiber constellations, a comparison of the tracking results of DSBT and SLT is included in this discussion of DSBT tracking results.

In the following evaluations the DSBT algorithm allows tenfold branching in the original seed voxel. In other voxels the branching is restricted to two. The simulation was, unless stated otherwise, evaluated on a subgrid of 33 voxels, including a margin of six voxels on all sides, the total subgrid covers a region of $15 \times 15 \times 1.6$ voxels ($\alpha = 0.1$) in the original data resolution. The FA threshold for the tracts was set to 0.35 (FA in the background is 0.3). A threshold of 0.8 was chosen for the tract smoothness (see section 7.1.1.1). The similarity threshold for the acceleration of the reconstruction was 0.5 for all simulated data sets, unless explicitly given otherwise. The simulation time was 0.001s, evaluated for 20 time steps.

The SLT results used to contrast the DSBT reconstructions were produced by DTI-Studio (v2.4). This program was not able to reconstruct tracts for ROIs with a fixed size of one voxel. The ROIs need to have a fixed size of two-by-two voxels inplane (XY) which is larger than the single voxel ROIs used by DSBT. The SLT algorithm considers every voxel in the dataset as a start for the reconstruction and reconstructs one tract per voxel. The results are then filtered with a selected ROI, so only tracts that connect to the ROI are included in the reconstruction. An example diffusion parameter file, containing all tracking parameters, is given in appendix B.

The coordinate of the ROI voxel for the DSBT evaluation is given as $\langle x, y, z \rangle$. The position of the ROI is given in Matlab coordinates which start from 1 instead of 0 (C++).

8.9.1. Branching

The simulated fiber in this data set consists of a branching fiber. Each arm of this fiber has an individual FA value as can be seen in Fig.8.21(a). The ROI was placed on the non-branching end of the fiber as shown in Fig.8.21(a). The reconstructed tracts are plotted in red over the FA map of the reconstructed fiber. The single voxel ROI for DSBT

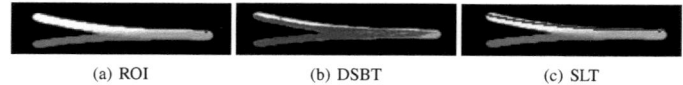

(a) ROI   (b) DSBT   (c) SLT

Figure 8.21.: *The tracking results for a simulated branching fiber.*

$\langle 134, 70, 8 \rangle$ lies completely inside of the two-by-two voxel ROI used by SLT. 8.21(b) gives the results for DSBT and 8.21(c) for SLT. The SLT results can only reconstruct one arm of the branching fiber with 81 tracts, whereas the DSBT algorithms reconstructs both arms with 3593 tracts.

The SLT tract is a straight line without any detail curving. The DSBT reconstruction is in general not as straight as the SLT results. The simulation results allow slight variations of the principal diffusion directions. The individual tracts can therefore be slightly curved. This also leads to wider reconstructed paths (see Fig.8.21(b)) because curving

8.9. Tracking Results

leads to detailed differences in the tracts and may therefore lead to more reconstructed tracts (not filtered by similarity threshold). The differences will accumulate along the tract path. In real data, fiber bundles are usually narrower than in the here evaluated synthetic data sets. The reconstruction should therefore not have room for much curving inside the fiber pathway, which is why the curving inside the tract is not considered a disadvantage.

8.9.1.1. Influence Of The Similarity Constraint

The similarity threshold causes one of two tracts whose differences are smaller than the given threshold to abort reconstruction (see also section 8.7.2). This pruning of the tracts will diminish the details in the reconstruction and improve the reconstruction time. Usually, the speedup outweighs the loss of detail but one needs to be aware of this tradeoff. The absolute number of cropped tracts is not important for the advantage. The earlier the tracts are cropped, the higher the speedup since each tract piece allows for m new tracts, with m the number of allowed branches. The gain is therefore $m^{\text{length}_{\text{uncut}} - \text{length}_{\text{cut}}} * reconstructionTime(tractPiece)$. The effect of the similarity

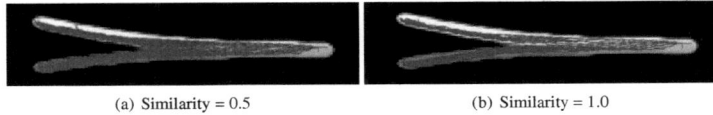

(a) Similarity = 0.5   (b) Similarity = 1.0

Figure 8.22.: *The influence of the similarity termination criterion on the reconstruction.*

threshold is illustrated on the comparison of an evaluation with a similarity threshold of 0.5 in Fig.8.22(a) and one with a threshold of 1.0 in Fig.:8.22(b). For the higher threshold the number of tracts is reduced as expected but still both arms of the branching tract are reconstructed. With a similarity threshold of 1.0 the reconstruction of 937 tracts (including 695 cropped ones) is complete in 2 hours and 41 minutes. With the reduced threshold of 0.5, the reconstruction of 3593 tracts (including 2346 cropped ones) takes 8 hours and 44 minutes. The trade off between the number of tracts, level of detail in the reconstruction, and speed needs to be considered on tuning this threshold.

8.9.1.2. The Influence Of The Subgrid Resolution

The influence of the subvoxel size, that is the reconstruction step length, on the results is illustrated on the example of the branching fiber in Fig.8.23. All results in presented in this figure used the same tracking parameters except for the subgrid resolution. The subgrid resolution determines how many subvoxels are contained in the subgrid of fixed size in the data domain. The larger the sub grid resolution, the smaller the subvoxels. The subvoxels influence the length of the reconstruction steps on the reconstructed tract pieces because the step is equal to the maximal subvoxel side length. All evaluations in

8. Diffusion Simulation Based Tracking

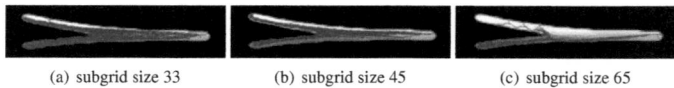

(a) subgrid size 33   (b) subgrid size 45   (c) subgrid size 65

Figure 8.23.: *The influence of the subvoxel size on the results illustrated on a simulated branching fiber.*

Fig.8.23 had a 6 subvoxel boundary surrounding the subgrid. For the tracking therefore only 21, 33 and 53 subvoxels were used.

The corresponding computation times for a single subgrid evaluation are 4.7s/0.005s, 14.9s/0.026s and 43.5s/0.117s for simulation/tract reconstruction. The evaluation takes longer for the higher resolution because more subvoxels need to be processed. The simulation takes only between $1.3e^{-4}$s and $1.6e^{-4}$s per subvoxel. There is no significant difference in the time required per subvoxel but the time required to process the same region in the data domain (one subgrid) varies considerably with the resolution.

The number of reconstructed tracts is diminished with increasing subgrid resolution. The reason for this is the interaction between subvoxel resolution and similarity constraint. With higher subvoxel resolution, the tracts are stopped by the same similarity threshold earlier, thereby preventing more tracts than clipping further along the reconstruction. The tracts on a high resolution subgrid are more similar because the points on the outermost front (the possible future seed points) lie closer together in the data domain because one subvoxel distance is less. A subvoxel in the isotropic subgrid resolution of 65 has size $0.23 \times 0.23 \times 0.025$ in the data domain, whereas the subgrid resolution of 33 generates subvoxels of size $0.45 \times 0.45 \times 0.049$. This causes the corresponding tract pieces to be closer to each other as well, rendering them more similar. The similarity constraint should therefore be tuned to match the subvoxel resolution of an evaluation. A high subgrid resolution should be matched with a low similarity threshold.

8.9.2. Orthogonal Crossing

This data set contains two fibers crossing at an 90 degree angle. Each fiber has an individual FA value. The ROIs for the evaluation are chosen on the ends of the fibers as illustrated in Fig.8.24(a). The ROIs for DSBT $\langle 134, 88, 8\rangle$ and $\langle 88, 134, 8\rangle$ are again completely inside the ROIs used for the SLT evaluation. The reconstructed horizontal tracts in the fiber with higher FA value (white in 8.24(a)) are plotted in red. The vertical tracts originating in the second ROI on the fiber with lower FA is plotted in green.

The SLT method returns 183 filtered tracts with both ROIs (135 in the horizontal fiber and 48 in the vertical one). DSBT reconstructs 158815 tracts in the horizontal fiber and 1534 in the vertical one.

The tracking along the vertical path (lower FA) with SLT stops in the region of fiber crossing, as shown in Fig.8.24(c). The eigenvector of the tensors in this region is dominated by the horizontal tract with the higher FA. This is also illustrated in Fig.7.2. The second order diffusion glyphs in this figure (ellipsoid) are colored according to the di-

8.9. Tracking Results

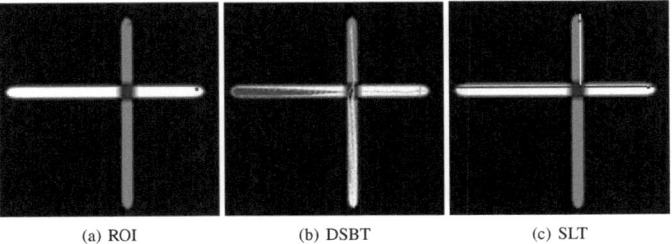

(a) ROI (b) DSBT (c) SLT

Figure 8.24.: *The tracking results for two orthogonally crossing fibers.*

rection of the corresponding principal eigenvector, red codes the horizontal orientation, green the vertical direction. The glyphs on the two tracts outside the intersection are very slim and cigar shaped. Approaching the region of crossing the effect of tensor averaging is clearly observable in the widening of the glyphs to a more spherical shape. In the intersection the dominance of the horizontal direction is only slight but clearly visible. This dominance allows the horizontal reconstruction to continue undisturbed. The smoothness conditions do not allow the tract to curve at a sharp angle, which is why the vertical tract stops and does not enter the horizontal fiber path.

DSBT reconstructs both fibers completely (see Fig.8.24(b)). This algorithm is not based on principal eigenvalues, therefore the dominance of the horizontal fiber does not prevent the reconstruction of the vertical tract. The green DSBT reconstruction of the vertical fiber with lower FA value fans out in the region of crossing. The fanning is caused by the dominance of the horizontal fiber. Without smoothness criteria the reconstruction would turn from the vertical fiber into the horizontal one as soon as it reaches the region that is horizontally dominated (center in Fig.7.2). The possible next diffusion seeds on the outermost diffusion front need to be smoothly connected to the current reconstruction to satisfy the smoothness criteria. Therefore, only slow curving tracts are possible. The path the tracts take across the region of crossing is ambiguous since the direction of the extrema of the diffusion fronts, the horizontal, is excluded by the smoothness criteria. The first few of the infinitely large number of points on the diffusion front with equal distance to the simulation seed, satisfying the smoothness criteria, are chosen as future simulation seeds. The front points with the same distance are ordered arbitrarily, the point selection is therefore not deterministic. In a region, such as the crossing in Fig.7.2, the details of the tracking results may differ but in a more global context the two individual fibers will always be reconstructed. The tracts do not require different FA values to be separable, opposed to the example reconstruction on a similar data set in [51].

8.9.3. Straight Crossing

In this data set two fibers with individual FA values cross at an angle smaller 40 degree. The ROIs are positioned at one end of each fiber as illustrated in Fig.8.25. The coordinates for the DSBT ROIs are $\langle 138, 91, 8 \rangle$ and $\langle 137, 57, 8 \rangle$. The tracts originating in the fiber with higher FA value are plotted in red and the ones reconstructing the fiber with lower FA in green over the corresponding FA map.

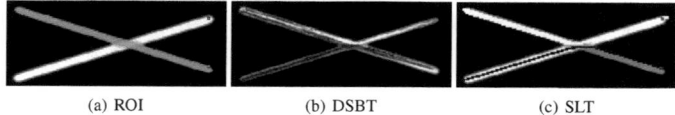

(a) ROI (b) DSBT (c) SLT

Figure 8.25.: *The tracking results for a straight crossing fibers.*

The SLT returns 228 tracts in total (18 red and 210 green). DSBT reconstructs 9626 red and 11785 green tratcs.

The smoothness criteria allow due to the small angle between the tracts a change of fibers (from one arm to the other) in the reconstruction. In Fig.8.25(c) both SLT reconstructions change the fiber in the region of crossing. No fiber is accurately reconstructed. The path of the SLT reconstructions can be explained with a look at the diffusion tensors in the crossing region (see Fig.8.26). The principal axis of the averaged tensors in the region of crossing is horizontal, this region can therefore only be traversed in left-right direction by the SLT method.

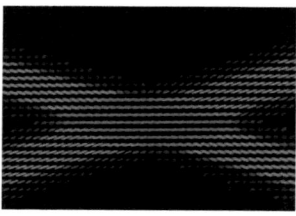

Figure 8.26.: *A detailed view of the tensors in the region of crossing. This plot was generated with the TensorViewer of the MedInria software package [29].*

In the DSBT reconstruction at least one fiber is reconstructed from beginning to end (see red tract in Fig.8.25(b)). The red tract is pushed toward the fiber with lower FA in the region of crossing because of the horizontal diffusion profile. A small portion of the reconstructed fiber bundles which are close to the second fiber in the intersection will branch into this fiber. The secondary branch is reconstructed until the fiber ends, leading to a false positive connection with the bottom-left fiber end. The fiber with the lower FA value is dominated in the region of crossing. The diffusion front is preferring the

8.9. Tracking Results

dominating fiber, therefore, the tract reconstruction that starts on the fiber with lower FA (green in Fig.8.25(b)) will follow the fiber with higher FA after the crossing region. The effect of the region of crossing is for DSBT not as dramatic as in the SLT reconstruction. The false positive reconstructions could be filtered with multiple ROIs similar to the brute force SLT approach shown in Fig.7.3 or with prior knowledge of the FA in the individual fibers [51].

8.9.4. Curve Crossing and Kissing

In this section two fiber constellations are discussed. One is a dataset consisting of two curving fibers which cross each other in a low angle. The other contains two curving fibers that touch each other in the center. Both fiber pairs contain two fibers with individual FA values.

The tensor profiles of these two cases are similar in the regions that contain both fibers. This kind of fiber constellation is therefore termed ambiguous because two interpretations of the tensor profiles (curved kissing and curved crossing fibers) are possible in the region the fibers touch. The ambiguousness of the tensor profiles can be seen in the tensor plots of both cases shown in Fig.8.27.

The FA map underlying the principal diffusion orientation (white lines) in Fig.8.27 are color coded (see section 4.2.1.3). Red indicates a horizontal orientation of the diffusion tensors. The background, where the FA is low in comparison no color coding is applied (the background is black). The differentiation between these two cases is very difficult for tracking algorithms. In both cases the merging tracts are represented by horizontal tensors in the region the fibers touch. The FA value is different for the individual fibers. They can, therefore, be visually distinguished in Fig.8.28(a) and 8.29(a).

The ROIs for the DSBT reconstruction for the curved crossing fibers are $\langle 130, 82, 8 \rangle$ and $\langle 122, 74, 8 \rangle$. The reconstructed plots for curved crossing fibers are for both reconstruction methods colored in green if they start in the fiber with higher FA and red if they start in the fiber with low FA. SLT returns 47 red reconstructed tracts and 13 green ones. DSBT reconstructs 236 red and 337 green tracts.

The curved crossing fibers cross at a small angle, a change in fibers is therefore, as discussed in section 8.9.3, possible without violation of the smoothness criteria. SLT is not able to reconstruct any fiber accurately in this constellation. The dominant fiber will change into the minor one after the overlapping region. The SLT result resembles a kissing fiber constellation more than a crossing one.

DSBT reconstructs both fibers. Both fibers branch after the region of crossing resulting in a false positive for each tract that could to be filtered with additional ROIs.

The ROIs for the DSBT reconstruction of the kissing fiber data set are $\langle 140, 69, 8 \rangle$ and $\langle 140, 86, 8 \rangle$. The reconstructed plots for curved crossing fibers are for both reconstruction methods plotted red if they start in the fiber with higher FA and green if they start in the fiber with low FA. The SLT method returns 63 red tracts and 3 green ones. DSBT is able to reconstruct 3852 red and 2342 green tracts.

For the kissing fiber data set the dominant fiber (higher FA, red tract) in Fig.8.29 is accurately reconstructed with both tracking methods. The minor fiber (green tract) is not

8. Diffusion Simulation Based Tracking

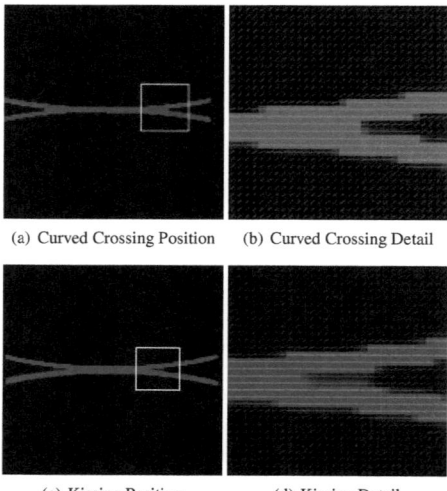

(a) Curved Crossing Position (b) Curved Crossing Detail

(c) Kissing Position (d) Kissing Detail

Figure 8.27.: *Curved crossing and kissing fibers have an ambiguous tensor profile. The first column gives the position of the detailed plots in the second column in the data set. The plots were created with the Camino software [21].*

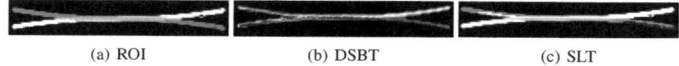

(a) ROI (b) DSBT (c) SLT

Figure 8.28.: *The tracking results for curved crossing fibers.*

completely reconstructed by SLT.

In contrast, DSBT is able to reconstruct both fibers completely. The minor fiber will split as the fibers are dividing again on the left of the plot. Some part of the green tract will falsely follow the dominant fiber with higher FA, resulting in a false positive reconstruction. This false positive can again be filtered by application of an additional ROI for the green tract. The dominant fiber is accurately reconstructed by the red tract.

The ambiguity of the kissing and curved crossing fiber cannot be resolved by DSBT but the fibers are opposed to the SLT reconstruction, both reconstructed in both cases. The low angle between the two fibers allows for branching of the tracts into both fibers in the region of crossing. The resulting false positives need to be removed by filtering with destination ROIs.

8.9. Tracking Results

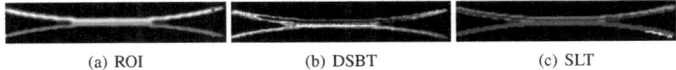

Figure 8.29.: *The tracking results for a kissing set of fibers.*

8.9.5. Spiral

The last data set explored here contains a single spiraling fiber with high FA value. The chosen ROI for DSBT is $\langle 129, 61, 8 \rangle$ as shown in Fig.8.30(a). Reconstructed tracts are plotted red for both reconstruction methods. SLT returns 193 tracts for the chosen ROI.

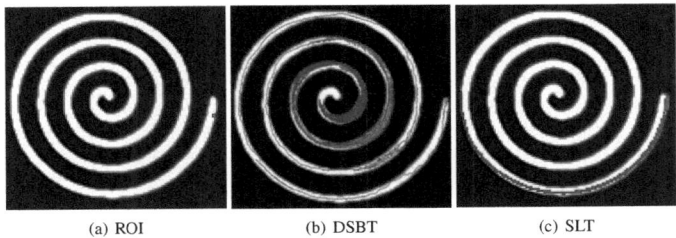

Figure 8.30.: *The tracking results for a spiraling fiber.*

DSBT reconstructs 23391 tracts.

Spiraling tracts are especially problematic for SLT. The curving is not accurately reconstructed by this method. The SLT reconstruction stops after half a turn, as shown in Fig.8.30(c). The length of the reconstruction is always half a turn, independent of where tracking is started on the spiral. The abortion of the tract results from a continuous drift toward the outside of the fiber pathway. SLT is not able to follow the relatively high curvature of the fiber with its discrete reconstruction steps.

The DSBT reconstruction has less problems with the reconstruction and follows the fiber further, as shown in Fig.8.30(b). The reconstruction did use an isotropic subgrid resolution of 45 with a border of 12 subvoxels. There is no tendency to drift observably and the spiral is reconstructed to the end. In the very end of the spiral, the random tensor orientations prohibit further reconstruction as illustrated in the tensor plot in Fig.8.31. The diffusion tensors are here depicted as cubes, the side lengths correspond to the eigenvalues. In the innermost turn the discrete tensor resolution is not able to follow the strong curving fiber, so the very end of the fiber cannot be reached by the reconstruction.

8.9.6. Conclusion from the Comparison

The tracts that were reconstructed with DSBT curve more than the straight lined SLT reconstructions. In my evaluation I considered a tract to be of good quality if it did

8. Diffusion Simulation Based Tracking

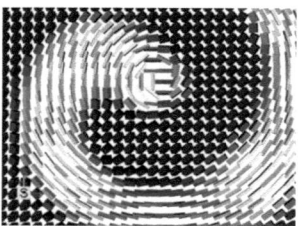

Figure 8.31.: *The tensor glyphs of the inner end of the spiral tract show a random orientation that prevents further reconstruction. This plot was generated with the TensorViewer of the MedInria software package [29].*

reach the end of the synthetic fiber because no formal tract quality measures are known from literature. Opposed to the SLT reconstruction, the DSBT reconstruction reaches both ends of the branching fiber. It is therefore considered superior. DSBT also handles curving and crossing fibers better than SLT. The quality of the reconstruction for crossing fibers is largely dependent on the angle between the fibers. A relatively small angle will lead to false positive reconstructions for DSBT, whereas the reconstruction fails completely in SLT (not one fiber is accurately reconstructed, see Fig.8.25(b)). False positives for DSBT means that the reconstruction might follow all of the arms from the region of crossing. By application of additional ROIs the problem of false positives can be resolved. The false positives are therefore not considered grave enough to negate the correct reconstruction (in red) of one of the straight crossing fibers. The application of filtering ROIs is common practice in fiber tracking. The reason why DSBT is able to resolve the problematic regions where SLT fails is that it takes a larger neighborhood into account when the direction for the next step is calculated. The neighborhood information keeps the reconstruction from deviating from the fiber in regions of crossing and allows smoother curving in the spiral fiber. A disadvantage for the DSBT is the large number of required computations which translates into longer evaluation time. The considerable improvement in the reconstruction warrants the investigation of further possibilities to speed up the TOA map based DSBT method.

8.9.7. Discussions

In this section I would like to discuss possible interpretations of the tracking results and possible extensions to more advanced diffusion models.

Probabilistic Interpretation of the Results

The results of a DSBT reconstruction can also be interpreted in a probabilistic context. Similar to probabilistic tracking algorithms known from literature (see section 7.1.2).

8.9. Tracking Results

The number of reconstructed tracts connecting a data point to the ROI gives a measure for the support of this connection by the data. To get a probability measure the number of tracts connecting a point with the seed point is divided by the total number of reconstructed tracts.

Cropping of the tracts especially with the similarity measure (see section 8.7.2) will influence the number of tracts passing through a voxel. The number of cropped tracts, whose similar tract connects the investigated point to the ROI, needs to be added to the tract count to establish the support for a connection.

Extending DSBT For Advanced Diffusion Models

As shown in section 4.3, new diffusion representations and models were recently developed to improve the handling of non-Gaussian diffusion in voxels that contain multiple fiber populations. The superior modeling of diffusion suggests that more accurate tracking results could be derived from these models. Some attempts have been made to do fiber tracking using advanced diffusion representation (see for example [18]).

My DSBT algorithm is based on a simulation of diffusion, the actual reconstruction works only on the TOA maps. This algorithm will therefore reconstruct tracts from any simulation result. I started exploring a simulation that uses more than the diffusion tensor information [Mang08].

The basic idea for our approach is based on an ADC interpretation of diffusion. We do not attempt to model the diffusion prior to the simulation, instead the ADC is computed for each measured gradient encoding direction (4.1). These ADC values give the strength of the diffusion in the corresponding directions. The ADCs for the individual gradient directions are interpolated to generate a set of ADCs that corresponds to a fixed equidistribution of directions used in the evaluation. This set of ADCs is computed for each voxel in the measured data set and is used to determine the particle flux in the data points. The resulting diffusion can be asymmetric (see Fig.8.32). Branching fibers should therefore be resolvable even in single voxels. The interpolation is performed with finite differences as illustrated in Fig.8.32. The approximation of the flux for the multi-directional case of HARDI data sets is a direct extension of (8.6). The approximated flux is given by:

$$\frac{\partial u_c}{\partial t} = k \sum_{d=1}^{N_d} \frac{[ADC_f(u_f - u_c)] - [ADC_b(u_c - u_b)]}{h_d^2}. \tag{8.9}$$

u is the particle concentration in a certain point, k is a constant scaling factor, d is the direction index and N_d is the number of evaluated directions. u_f and u_b are computed by linear interpolation of the concentration values of the neighboring points (along the green lines in Fig.8.32). ADC_f is the interpolation of the ADCs in the evaluated direction d in point c and the point corresponding to u_f. The ADC corresponding to u_f is generated by linear interpolation of the ADC values in the neighboring grid points (along the green lines in Fig.8.32). ADC_b is similarly defined. The simulated diffusion is allowed to be asymmetric since ADC_f and ADC_b need not be equal, opposed to the measured ADCs. The ADCs for the gradient direction (gray dotted line) are illustrated as red arrows of

8. Diffusion Simulation Based Tracking

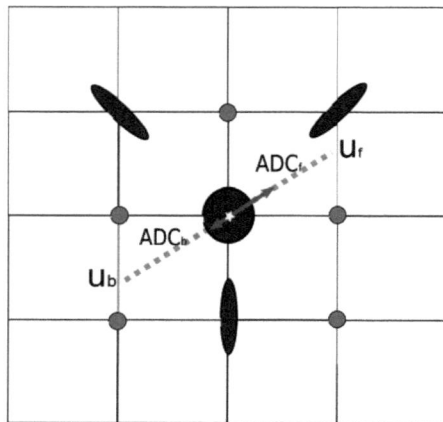

Figure 8.32.: *The interpolations needed for the more advanced diffusion simulation are illustrated here in a 2D scheme for one exemplary gradient direction d. The flux (8.9) is estimated for the point in the center, marked with a yellow star. The points on the fiber are given in blue, the ones on the background in orange. The 2D diffusion ellipsoid, corresponding to the second order diffusion tensor, illustrates the corresponding (Gaussian) diffusion profiles. The ADCs, corresponding to direction d (ADC_f), and $-d$ (ADC_b) are illustrated with red arrows. They are computed by linear interpolation, first between neighboring data points along the green lines, and then along the gray dotted line.*

different length in Fig.8.32.

The lack of modeling in this simulation approach is both risk and chance. As previously mentioned in the ADC discussion (see section 4.1), the ADC is a combined representation of noise and signal. The simulation results might therefore be more susceptible to noise. Since the ADC values are interpolated some of the random noise should be canceled (see discussion of SNR in section 2.5.1). The effect of noise might therefore not be very dramatic. The dependence of the tracking results on noise still needs to be determined in more elaborate evaluations.

9. Summary And Outlook

In this chapter I want to summarize my findings. The results are ordered according to their presentation in the previous text. In the second part of this chapter, open questions to the individual subjects are presented and discussed.

9.1. Summary

9.1.1. Higher Order Tensor Models

I could show that by estimating the even and the odd order tensors in the HOT hierarchy model [57] with separate equation systems, the minimal required number of encoding directions for the HOT hierarchy, up to a tensor order of four, could be reduced from 31 (6+10+15 independent tensor elements) to 21 (6+15 independent tensor elements). This reduces the number of required diffusion weighted measurements by over 30%. In addition, I showed that two b-factors are sufficient to estimate the tensors for this HOT hierarchy model. This reduced the required measurement time dramatically since the method was previously only published using 10 b-factors. The optimal choice of these two b-factors still needs to be determined.

The phase in EPI measurements is much too distorted to be of use for the HOT hierarchy estimation. But still the even order tensors only hierarchy is a useful tool for the investigation of heterodirectional voxels which contain multiple fiber orientations. Fiber crossings can be adequately resolved and the fiber orientation is accurately reconstructed opposed to the single HOT model [73].

9.1.2. Gradient Encoding Schemes

I showed that angular distance is not a good quality measure for GES quality. The evaluation of several quality measures from literature showed that they are not suitable for the evaluation of GES quality for higher order tensor models. The b-factor dependence of quality measures, like the *condition number*, render a direct comparison between higher order tensor models impossible because the HOT hierarchy requires, opposed to the single HOT model, at least two b-factors greater zero (when a low number of encoding directions (smaller 200 [57]) is used. The choice of the b-factors can gravely influence the b-factor dependent quality indices. For the HOT hierarchy, a interdependence between the two b-factors was observable. The single HOT model requires only one b-factor. The

9. Summary And Outlook

corresponding quality indices therefore change with the b-factor but the interdependence of the chosen b-factors is no problem for this model. The different uses of b-factors allow only intra model evaluation of the quality indices.

Different methods for the classification of GES were investigated, the most successful method was the evaluation of the *signal accuracy* in section 6.7. This method can be evaluated for all tensor models and is not only a tool for the classification of GES quality but can also be used to investigate the model accuracy. This method supports the results from all other evaluations, especially from the condition number evaluation (section 6.4) and the gravity distance (section 6.5). It disqualifies Cond, Ana1 and Ana2 as best possible general purpose GES.

The second order tensor evaluation of the GES quality by *classification of estimation quality* (section 6.6) showed that the ForceSingle GES is not well equipped for the second order tensor estimation with less than twelve directions. This scheme is therefore not a candidate for best all purpose GES.

My investigation of model accuracy shows the superiority of the Icosa and ForcePairs GES. Of these two, ForcePairs is the only GES that is able to generate an arbitrary number of equally well distributed encoding directions, which is an advantage if the number of directions needs to be minimized due to restrictions in the available measurement time. This practical advantage led to my decision to favor ForcePairs over Icosa.

9.1.3. Fibertracking

In chapter 8, I introduced a new fiber tracking method which is based on the simulation of diffusion and uses time-of-arrival maps to store the simulation results. I did show that practical limitations prohibit successful tractography with only one simulation process, even if a large number of simulation steps is evaluated (see section 8.5). One limiting factor is the concentration on the simulated diffusion front. The virtual concentration peak which will diffuse during the simulation process will get wider and shallower with each simulation time step. Since the background concentration value is due to the numerical solver never exactly zero, the diffusion front needs to be extracted by thresholding the concentration value. At one point, the concentration on the diffusion front will be indistinguishable from the background concentration, since the initial peak has a limited hight. A second problem that occurs when DSBT tries to use only one large simulation is *bleeding* of the diffusion front through the background. For example, in the reconstruction of a tight U-shaped fiber starting in one leg of the U, the second leg can be reached by diffusion which courses through the background (low FA) faster than by the one following the U-shape. This leads to problems in the reconstruction (see Fig.8.11) because the TOA and therefore the gradients will be faulty (not correspond to the course of the fiber) in these regions of bleeding. To overcome the problem with single simulation DSBT, I chose a series of successive simulations to reconstruct the tracts. The simulation process is evaluated on a given subgrid. All steps of DSBT (simulation, TOA map generation and gradient descend) are performed on this subgrid and the endpoints of the so reconstructed tract pieces are used as future simulation seeds. The individual tract pieces are smoothly connected at their fusion points (end = future seed). This restriction

9.1. Summary

to a smaller evaluation region reduces the effects caused by *bleeding* and render a initial concentration peak with limited hight sufficient.

This implementation of DSBT is very time consuming. One of the reasons for this is that each simulation step requires several seconds computation time. The reduction of the subgrid resolution accelerates the computation time because the amount of subvoxels that need to be handled in a single simulation is reduced. This reduction, on the other hand, results in larger reconstruction steps because of the increased suboxel size.

An advantage of DSBT is that it allows branching of the tract in each simulation. The number of tracts and therefore the number of simulations increases exponentially (c^s, with c the number of allowed branches and s the number of steps).

Since the simulations are the most time consuming part of DSBT, I explored several criteria for the reduction of tract pieces and thereby simulations (see section 8.7.2 and 8.7.3). The simulation cannot be replaced by computationally cheaper second order diffusion propagator methods (see section 8.7.5) since this would reduce DSBT to a streamline technique. I could successfully apply a similarity criterion to accelerate the reconstruction (see section 8.7.2). This criterion will terminate the reconstruction in a tract if its deviation from a previously reconstructed tract is smaller than a chosen threshold. If extensive investigations are to be performed on a data set, a look-up-table (LUT) containing the TOA maps can be generated to avoid computationally expensive simulation during the investigation (see section 8.7.4). The computation of the LUT is expensive and therefore only advantageous for extensive investigations of several fiber populations.

I could show, on the results from synthetic fiber tracts, that DSBT is able to resolve complicated fiber constellations. Especially curving, crossing and branching tracts are resolvable with DSBT (see section 8.9). In the comparison with SLT results, the improvement of the reconstruction with DSBT becomes more clear. SLT has, especially with crossing and curving fibers, considerable problems which can be nicely resolved with DSBT. The advantages in the reconstruction warrant further investigations to optimize the speed of the evaluation. Especially parallel processing promises further speedup.

Fibers crossing in a small angle might cause branching in the reconstructed tracts. The branches will follow every possible fiber direction, causing false reconstructions. These false positive connections can be filtered by application of additional ROIs. The accurate reconstruction in these complicated cases therefore needs some prior knowledge but is still an improvement to SLT.

A particularly interesting field of research in the context of fiber tracking is tracking on advanced diffusion representations or models (see for example section 4.3). DSBT has the great advantage that the actual tracking is performed on simulation results, therefore, if a diffusion simulation can be performed on the advanced diffusion data, DSBT can be used for tracking on the data. More accurate diffusion representation promises more accurate simulation results and therefore more accurate tracking. In chapter 8.9.7, I discuss a first approach for a more advanced simulation.

9.2. Open Questions

9.2.1. Higher Order Tensor Models

HOT evaluations promise to be valuable for more advanced diffusion evaluations. Especially the HOT hierarchy [57] is promising. But the question which b-factors should be used is still under investigation. I could show that at least two b-factors should be used for this model but could not yet determine which b-factors are optimal.

Another question regarding the HOT hierarchy is the measurability of the phase information. Especially in EPI the phase is too distorted to be used in the HOT hierarchy. The question whether more advanced measurement techniques such as SNAILS [60] could be used to measure the phase information with sufficient quality is still under investigation. But even the even order HOT hierarchy (without odd order tensors and therefore without phase information) is a useful tool to evaluate fiber crossings, since these are resolvable by even order and the orientation of the fibers is accurately represented, opposed to the single HOT model [59].

To be usable in a clinical environment, it would be good to be able to extract the important information from the HOT hierarchy and display them in scalar maps, similar to, for example, the FA maps that are derived from the second order tensor model [Liu07]. For some of the higher order tensors diagonalizations have been proposed to compute the eigenvalues. The interpretation of these higher order eigenvalues is currently not clear, which makes the interpretation of eigenvalue based scalar measures impossible. The usability of other scalar values which are based on, for example, the shape of the PDF is still under investigation.

9.2.2. Gradient Encoding Schemes

I showed in the second order evaluation (see section 6.6) that the improvement resulting from more than 30 gradient encoding directions for this model does not warrant the additional measurement time. The findings are in accordance with Jones [47] who showed a similar result for the ForcePairs GES only. The question whether the higher order tensors have an preferred number of encoding directions and if so what number should be chosen needs to be further investigated.

At the moment, no universal quality measure for GES is available. The *evaluation of the signal accuracy* (see section 6.7) could be used as such. An optimal set of tensors or fiber constellations should be defined to be able to use the signal accuracy evaluation in a standardized fashion. This should make an objective evaluation of GES and diffusion models possible.

9.2.3. Fibertracking

To be usable in clinical context, the DSBT tracking algorithm needs to be faster. I showed that the algorithm is able to resolve synthetic fiber constellations that present unsolvable

9.2. Open Questions

problems for commonly used SLT methods (see section 8.9). Improving the reconstruction speed for DSBT is therefore a worthy goal. Parallel processing, for example, could be used to speedup the computation.

The question how earlier anisotropy thresholding (before or during the simulation process) affects the simulation results needs to be investigated. If the results are not affected in a negative way, the early thresholding might lead to an improvement in computation time because more isotropic diffusion tensors (the ones that are artificially set to zero) occur in the evaluation.

Different approaches to define a simulation on advanced diffusion representations need to be evaluated. In section 8.9.7, I discussed a first simple method. More advanced methods should be able to further improve the tracking results.

The possibility to use a propagator corresponding to an advanced diffusion representation instead of a diffusion simulation needs to be evaluated. This method might present a way to use advanced diffusion models in DSBT without the need to define new simulation methods.

A formal quality criterion for the classification and comparison of fiber tracts would be desirable. I proposed a crude measure on synthetic data sets that considers a reconstruction successful if the fiber was completely reconstructed (end to end). This quality measure clearly needs refinement. The question whether curving tracts are inferior to straight ones is for example not taken into account. This approach to measure quality is also only applicable to synthetic fiber reconstruction where the start and end of a fiber is known.

A. Tables With Results From GES-Evaluation

This chapter contains tables with the actual condition number evaluation results discussed in chapter 5. The discussion in this chapter was mainly supported by figures illustrating the data in the following tables. The detailed tables are supplied to allow the interested reader to explore the data by himself.

First, the results for the standard second order tensor are presented in Tab. A.1. More

N_e	Ana1	Ana2	Cond	Icosa	ForceSingle	ForcePairs
15	7.7641	1.7201	1.6870	1.5811	1.5992	1.5939
16	2.9924	1.6914	1.6878	1.5811	1.5903	1.5812
21	2.4863	1.6727	1.6880	1.5811	1.6022	1.5811
30	2.7475	1.6251	1.6924	1.5811	1.5878	1.5846
46	1.7755	1.6056	1.6937	1.5811	1.5838	1.5811
81	1.6429	1.5928	1.6950	1.5811	1.5818	1.5815
126	1.7711	1.5881	1.6942	1.5811	1.5818	1.5816

Table A.1.: *The mean condition number evaluated for the second order tensor.*

detailed information can be gathered from the minimal and maximal condition number encountered in the rotational dependent evaluation. This additional information is given in Tab. A.2 and A.3.

N_e	Ana1			Ana2			Cond		
	max	min	mean	max	min	mean	max	min	mean
15	8.395	6.510	7.764	1.892	1.631	1.720	2.001	1.335	1.687
16	3.625	2.169	2.992	1.815	1.630	1.691	2.009	1.338	1.688
21	2.931	1.858	2.486	1.802	1.631	1.673	1.990	1.330	1.688
30	2.939	2.255	2.748	1.655	1.609	1.625	2.002	1.326	1.692
46	1.915	1.599	1.776	1.630	1.600	1.606	1.999	1.324	1.694
81	1.731	1.599	1.643	1.600	1.591	1.593	2.000	1.323	1.695
126	1.889	1.672	1.771	1.591	1.588	1.588	1.999	1.324	1.694

Table A.2.: *The condition number evaluated for the second order tensor.*

N_e	Icosa			ForceSingle			ForcePairs		
	max	min	mean	max	min	mean	max	min	mean
15	1.581	1.581	1.581	1.633	1.546	1.599	1.603	1.560	1.594
16	1.581	1.581	1.581	1.602	1.581	1.590	1.581	1.581	1.581
21	1.581	1.581	1.581	1.619	1.591	1.602	1.581	1.581	1.581
30	1.581	1.581	1.581	1.589	1.586	1.588	1.588	1.573	1.585
46	1.581	1.581	1.581	1.586	1.583	1.584	1.581	1.581	1.581
81	1.581	1.581	1.581	1.582	1.581	1.582	1.582	1.580	1.582
126	1.581	1.581	1.581	1.583	1.582	1.582	1.583	1.581	1.582

Table A.3.: *The condition number evaluated for the second order tensor (continued).*

After the second order tensor the higher order tensors for both the single HOT and the HOT hierarchy model are presented. For the higher order evaluations only the detailed tables containing the minimal and maximal as well as the mean condition number are given.

N_e	Ana1			Ana2			Cond		
	max	min	mean	max	min	mean	max	min	mean
15	-	-	-	-	-	-	146.53	68.50	98.89
16	-	-	-	73.20	56.71	63.07	140.90	64.09	91.58
21	25.74	11.21	16.69	29.36	22.31	24.82	74.50	27.61	42.12
30	16.72	10.14	12.10	5.26	3.84	4.39	15.13	8.26	11.31
46	7.08	4.46	6.23	4.00	3.59	3.74	8.99	3.90	6.26
81	4.93	3.69	4.12	3.84	3.63	3.71	9.93	3.40	6.40
126	5.20	3.70	4.28	3.79	3.67	3.72	8.12	2.96	5.20

Table A.4.: *The condition number evaluated for the fourth order single HOT model.*

A. Tables With Results From GES-Evaluation

N_e	Icosa			ForceSingle			ForcePairs		
	max	min	mean	max	min	mean	max	min	mean
15	5.35	4.08	4.95	8771.09	5521.51	6848.44	4.74	3.81	4.37
16	7.44	6.19	6.85	16917.09	12476.68	14083.18	3.79	3.75	3.76
21	3.85	3.79	3.81	44.10	32.03	39.45	3.85	3.79	3.81
30	3.88	3.81	3.83	3.93	3.61	3.75	3.79	3.71	3.75
46	3.85	3.79	3.81	3.81	3.71	3.75	3.77	3.74	3.75
81	3.79	3.75	3.77	3.76	3.73	3.75	3.76	3.74	3.75
126	3.84	3.79	3.81	3.76	3.74	3.75	3.75	3.74	3.75

Table A.5.: *The condition number evaluated for the fourth order single HOT model.*

N_e	Ana1			Ana2		
	max	min	mean	max	min	mean
21	973936	566689	843736	603460	510643	540383
30	1084100	701624	902154	546500	483532	501999
46	682398	470225	600551	514631	485427	492376
81	550847	506203	523415	497680	485537	488312
126	610028	514886	555034	491764	485533	486987

Table A.6.: *The condition number evaluated for the fourth order HOT hierarchy (even order estimation matrix).*

N_e	Cond			Icosa		
	max	min	mean	max	min	mean
21	1918078	831798	1285663	499044	484104	489747
30	1028004	534892	770927	503308	483747	492999
46	1025588	433263	691815	498680	484135	489616
81	1102011	416280	740454	490279	484850	486702
126	1063696	438137	703462	498055	484188	489392

Table A.7.: *The condition number evaluated for the fourth order HOT hierarchy (continued).*

N_e	ForceSingle			ForcePairs		
	max	min	mean	max	min	mean
21	535887	505818	526518	499022	484114	489822
30	494302	489012	491882	489924	480836	487031
46	488038	486056	487270	487199	485233	485817
81	486115	485413	485867	486150	484974	485524
126	486145	485513	485735	486160	485300	485641

Table A.8.: *The condition number evaluated for the fourth order HOT hierarchy (continued).*

N_e	Ana1			Ana2			Cond		
	max	min	mean	max	min	mean	max	min	mean
30	-	-	-	218.5	126.9	172.0	3719.2	1237.2	2192.2
46	40.0	17.2	30.2	25.1	17.1	20.8	172.1	36.5	81.3
81	18.6	11.8	14.8	10.5	9.8	9.9	88.8	14.0	42.3
126	14.7	10.7	12.4	10.1	9.8	9.9	57.3	11.4	31.2

Table A.9.: *The condition number evaluated for the sixth order single HOT model.*

N_e	Icosa			ForceSingle			ForcePairs		
	max	min	mean	max	min	mean	max	min	mean
30	-	-	-	39831.4	22262.6	28134.3	11.0	9.7	10.3
46	10.5	9.9	10.2	42.6	33.5	38.1	10.1	9.9	10.01
81	10.2	9.7	10.0	10.0	9.8	9.9	9.9	9.8	9.9
126	10.4	9.7	10.2	9.9	9.8	9.8	9.9	9.9	9.9

Table A.10.: *The condition number evaluated for the sixth order single HOT model (continued).*

N_e	Ana1			Ana2		
	max	min	mean	max	min	mean
81	201.8E+9	174.7E+9	193.3E+9	179.1E+9	176.2E+9	176.9E+9
126	224.5E+9	187.3E+9	201.8E+9	177.6E+9	176.4E+9	176.6E+9

Table A.11.: *The condition number evaluated for the sixth order HOT hierarchy (even order estimation matrix).*

N_e	Cond			Icosa		
	max	min	mean	max	min	mean
81	843.4E+9	180.4E+9	477.2E+9	180.4E+9	173.3E+9	177.1E+9
126	104.2E+10	206.5E+9	512.0E+9	185.4E+9	171.0E+9	178.0E+9

Table A.12.: *The condition number evaluated for the sixth order HOT hierarchy (continued).*

N_e	Cond			Icosa		
	max	min	mean	max	min	mean
81	177.4E+9	176.5E+9	177.0E+9	177.0E+9	176.3E+9	176.6E+9
126	177.1E+9	176.3E+9	176.8E+9	177.0E+9	176.4E+9	176.7E+9

Table A.13.: *The condition number evaluated for the sixth order HOT hierarchy (continued).*

A. Tables With Results From GES-Evaluation

N_e	Ana1			Ana2		
	max	min	mean	max	min	mean
46	840E+17	679E+14	482E+15	18487	10169	15487
81	431	237	317	385	248	355
126	311	184	268	162	150	158

Table A.14.: *The condition number evaluated for the eighth order single HOT model.*

N_e	Cond			Icosa		
	max	min	mean	max	min	mean
46	83462	25669	53426	192	172	186
81	8474	5591	7103	156	150	153
126	6740	1309	4420	158	148	154

Table A.15.: *The condition number evaluated for the eighth order single HOT model (continued).*

N_e	ForceSingle			ForcePairs		
	max	min	mean	max	min	mean
46	47240	36002	40128	190	176	182
81	577	409	505	154	150	151
126	152	150	151	150	149	149

Table A.16.: *The condition number evaluated for the eighth order single HOT model.*

B. DTI-Studio Evaluation Parameters

Here the parameter file used in the diffusion evaluation in section 8.9 is given. Only the input image file (*InputImgFile*) needed to be customized for the individual data sets. The ROIs could not be stored but needed to be drawn by hand individually.

```
//--- Begin of ".dpf" file ---//
Begin
ImageWidth:   150
ImageHeight:  150
ImageSlices:  16

ProcSliceStart: 0
ProcSliceEnd:   15

FieldOfView(X): 150
FieldOfView(Y): 150

// PixelSize(X): 0.9766   //This is an optional field
// PixelSize(Y): 0.9766

SliceThickness: 1

B-Value: 1000

Begin_Of_Gradient_Table
 1:  0,             0,             0
 2:  1.0000000e+00,  0.0000000e+00,  0.0000000e+00
 3:  1.6602059e-01,  9.8612229e-01,  0.0000000e+00
 4: -1.0996723e-01,  6.6380222e-01,  7.3977958e-01
 5:  9.0124247e-01, -4.1911276e-01, -1.1002960e-01
 6: -1.6902341e-01, -6.0108326e-01,  7.8110819e-01
 7: -8.1471083e-01, -3.8586304e-01,  4.3284637e-01
 8:  6.5603543e-01,  3.6601977e-01,  6.6003564e-01
 9:  5.8224081e-01,  8.0033101e-01,  1.4305917e-01
10:  9.0018861e-01,  2.5905428e-01,  3.5007335e-01
11:  6.9329922e-01, -6.9830138e-01,  1.7807686e-01
```

B. DTI-Studio Evaluation Parameters

```
12:   3.5685283e-01,  -9.2361909e-01,  -1.3994229e-01
13:   5.4314069e-01,  -4.8812644e-01,  -6.8317697e-01
14:  -5.2514443e-01,  -3.9610894e-01,   7.5320716e-01
15:  -6.3921641e-01,   6.8923334e-01,   3.4111549e-01
16:  -3.2996618e-01,  -1.2998668e-02,  -9.4390325e-01
17:  -5.2402882e-01,  -7.8304307e-01,   3.3501843e-01
18:   6.0876050e-01,  -6.4974438e-02,  -7.9068893e-01
19:   2.2005524e-01,  -2.3305851e-01,  -9.4723779e-01
20:  -3.9993182e-03,  -9.0984488e-01,  -4.1492926e-01
21:  -5.1070107e-01,   6.2663321e-01,  -5.8865544e-01
22:   4.1383657e-01,   7.3670906e-01,   5.3478880e-01
23:  -6.7893109e-01,   1.3898589e-01,  -7.2092683e-01
24:   8.8394873e-01,  -2.9598283e-01,   3.6197901e-01
25:   2.6199515e-01,   4.3199201e-01,   8.6298403e-01
26:   8.7981966e-02,   1.8496209e-01,  -9.7879937e-01
27:   2.9395753e-01,  -9.0686897e-01,   3.0195637e-01
28:   8.8704480e-01,  -8.9004495e-02,  -4.5302288e-01
29:   2.5697700e-01,  -4.4296036e-01,   8.5892313e-01
30:   8.5992863e-02,   8.6692805e-01,  -4.9095925e-01
31:   8.6325470e-01,   5.0414875e-01,  -2.5007378e-02

End_Of_Gradient_Table

InputImgFile: C:\DICOM_DTIStudio\KissingREC

InputImgOrder: Gradient_By_Gradient
// Slice_By_Slice or Gradient_By_Gradient
End
//--- End of ".dpf" file ---//
```

In the tensor estimation a background threshold of ten was chosen all other parameters were set to default. The tracking allowed a curvature of 70 degrees. The FA threshold used in the tracking was 0.35 equal to the FA value used by DSBT.

C. Input Tensors For Simulations

Here the tensors used in the simulations in section 6 are given.

C.1. Second Order Tensors

These tensors were used in section 6.6.

The cigar shaped tensor:
$$\begin{pmatrix} 2e-3 & -6.88e-7 & 2.06e-6 \\ -6.88e-7 & 0.231e-3 & 1.43e-6 \\ 2.06e-6 & 1.43e-6 & 0.231e-3 \end{pmatrix}.$$

The oblate shaped tensor:
$$\begin{pmatrix} 2e-3 & -1.3737e-6 & 1.3748e-6 \\ -1.3737e-6 & 1.1154e-3 & 8.8522e-4 \\ 1.3748e-6 & 8.8522e-4 & 1.1141e-3 \end{pmatrix}.$$

C.2. HOT Hierarchy Tensors

The tensors for the HOT hierarchy up to order four for a voxel containing two orthogonal crossing fibers. These tensors are used in section 6.7.

The second order tensor D_{ij}:
$$\begin{pmatrix} 0.0014 & -1.1839e-6 & -1.3729e-6 \\ -1.1839e-6 & 0.0014 & 3.9717e-7 \\ -1.3729e-6 & 3.9717e-7 & 2.2957e-4 \end{pmatrix}.$$

The third order tensor $D_{i,j,k}$:

$k = 1:$ $\begin{pmatrix} -0.0066e-7 & 0.0323e-7 & -0.0557e-7 \\ 0.0323e-7 & -0.1173e-7 & 0.0439e-7 \\ -0.0557e-7 & 0.0439e-7 & 0.0236e-7 \end{pmatrix},$

$k = 2:$ $\begin{pmatrix} 0.0323e-7 & -0.1173e-7 & 0.0439e-7 \\ -0.1173e-7 & 0.0704e-7 & 0.0678e-7 \\ 0.0439e-7 & 0.0678e-7 & -0.0499e-7 \end{pmatrix},$

C. Input Tensors For Simulations

$$k = 3: \begin{pmatrix} -0.0557e-7 & 0.0439e-7 & 0.0236e-7 \\ 0.0439e-7 & 0.0678e-7 & -0.0499e-7 \\ 0.0236e-7 & -0.0499e-7 & 0.2180e-7 \end{pmatrix}.$$

The fourth order tensor $D_{i,j,k,l}$:

$$k = 1 \text{ and } l = 1: 1.0e-8 * \begin{pmatrix} 0.7409 & 0.0001 & -0.0036 \\ 0.0001 & -0.0950 & 0.0011 \\ -0.0036 & 0.0011 & 0.0073 \end{pmatrix},$$

$$k = 2 \text{ and } l = 1: 1.0e-9 * \begin{pmatrix} 0.0014 & -0.9503 & 0.0106 \\ -0.9503 & -0.0033 & -0.0147 \\ 0.0106 & -0.0147 & -0.0038 \end{pmatrix},$$

$$k = 3 \text{ and } l = 1: 1.0e-10 * \begin{pmatrix} -0.3638 & 0.1062 & 0.7338 \\ 0.1062 & -0.1468 & -0.0383 \\ 0.7338 & -0.0383 & -0.0132 \end{pmatrix},$$

$$k = 1 \text{ and } l = 2: 1.0e-9 * \begin{pmatrix} 0.0014 & -0.9503 & 0 \\ -0.9503 & -0.0033 & -0.0147 \\ 0.0106 & -0.0147 & -0.0038 \end{pmatrix},$$

$$k = 2 \text{ and } l = 2: 1.0e-8 * \begin{pmatrix} -0.0950 & -0.0003 & -0.0015 \\ -0.0003 & 0.7283 & 0.0010 \\ -0.0015 & 0.0010 & 0.0067 \end{pmatrix},$$

$$k = 3 \text{ and } l = 2: 1.0e-10 * \begin{pmatrix} 0.1062 & -0.1468 & -0.0383 \\ -0.1468 & 0.1006 & 0.6670 \\ 0 & 0.6670 & -0.1031 \end{pmatrix},$$

$$k = 1 \text{ and } l = 3: 1.0e-10 * \begin{pmatrix} -0.3638 & 0.1062 & 0.7338 \\ 0.1062 & -0.1468 & -0.0383 \\ 0.7338 & -0.0383 & -0.0132 \end{pmatrix},$$

$$k = 2 \text{ and } l = 3: 1.0e-10 * \begin{pmatrix} 0.1062 & -0.1468 & -0.0383 \\ 0 & 0.1006 & 0.6670 \\ -0.0383 & 0.6670 & -0.1031 \end{pmatrix},$$

$$k = 3 \text{ and } l = 3: 1.0e-10 * \begin{pmatrix} 0.7338 & -0.0383 & -0.0132 \\ -0.0383 & 0.6670 & -0.1031 \\ -0.0132 & -0.1031 & 0.0555 \end{pmatrix},$$

D. The Relationship Between The ADC Glyph And The Reynold Tensor Glyph

The ADC glyph described in section 4.1 has the shape of a peanut similar to the Reynolds tensor glyph presented in section 4.2.2. The Reynolds tensor glyph is derived by sampling the tensor $\mathbf{D}$ with a given number of unit vectors sampling a sphere. The radius r of the resulting glyph in the sampling points corresponding the the direction $\mathbf{g}$ is given by

$$r(\mathbf{g}) = \mathbf{g}\mathbf{D}\mathbf{g}^T. \tag{D.1}$$

The ADC is defined as $ln(S_\mathbf{g}/S_0)/-b)$, where S_0 is the unweighted image b is the diffusion weighting factor and $S_\mathbf{g}$ the diffusion weighted signal. With (4.2) the following equalities hold:

$$\begin{aligned}
S_\mathbf{g} &= S_0 exp(-b\mathbf{g}\mathbf{D}\mathbf{g}^T) \\
S_\mathbf{g}/S_0 &= exp(-b\mathbf{g}\mathbf{D}\mathbf{g}^T) \\
ln(S_\mathbf{g}/S_0) &= -b\mathbf{g}\mathbf{D}\mathbf{g}^T \\
ln(S_\mathbf{g}/S_0)/-b &= \mathbf{g}\mathbf{D}\mathbf{g}^T = ADC.
\end{aligned} \tag{D.2}$$

The definition of the direction dependent radius of the Reynolds tensor glyph (D.1) and the ADC are therefore the same.

In the case of noise free signal the ADC and the Reynolds tensor glyph are the same, otherwise, the ADC glyph is distorted. This distortion will cause the ADC glyph to deviate from the true peanut shape as illustrated in Fig.4.2. The sampling of the tensor in noisy data is distorted, therefore the shape is inaccurate. If the tensor is first fit to the noisy data and then represented by the Reynolds tensor glyph the surface will be smooth because the noise in the individual sampling directions is modeled by the tensor and not taken from the measurement directly.

E. List of Figures

2.1.	The two properties of a proton that are important for MRI are illustrated.	6
2.2.	The net magnetization flips into the XY-plane.	7
2.3.	The effect of linear gradient on the static magnetic field B_0. Illustration adopted from [67].	8
2.4.	Example images for the two main imaging contrasts.	10
2.5.	The stages of the magnetization in the image acquisition.	11
2.6.	A diagram depicting a simple spin echo sequence (image adopted from [36]).	12
2.7.	A diagram of the gradient echo sequence (image adopted from [36]). . .	13
2.8.	EPI sequence timing diagram with an echo train (image adopted from [36]).	14
2.9.	An example for PVE in a voxel with two kinds of matter.	17
3.1.	Coronal cut through the brain. The gray matter is the darker outermost region of the brain. It encloses the white matter. The brain surface is folded producing sulci (grooves) and gyri (elevations). Image adapted from [82].	19
3.2.	The anatomy of a neuron is illustrated in (a). The axon of a neuron is isolated by a myelin sheath that is wound tightly around the fiber as illustrated in a cut through the axon in (b). The illustrations were adapted from [89]	19
3.3.	The effect of diffusion wheighting on the signal. The illustration was addopted from [67].	22
3.4.	Pulsed gradient echo sequence for diffusion weighted imaging.	23
4.1.	An example ADC intensity map.	27
4.2.	ADC glyph for 81 gradient encoding directions.	28
4.3.	The symmetric tensor is illustrated. Each of the nine images gives the tensor elements, here visualized for a single slice in the data set. The off-diagonal images are mirrored on the diagonal. There are therefore only six different images (independent tensor elements). The signal in the diagonal tensor elements is stronger and less noisy than in the off-diagonal images.	29

List of Figures

4.4. The off-diagonal elements give the tilt of the diffusion glyph. This is illustrated in two 2D examples. The tensor elements are given in the subtext of the plots. 29

4.5. In this figure the advantage of color coding the directionality of the measured diffusion information in a scalar diffusion index is illustrated on the example of FA maps. The FA is a scalar value that is usually visualized as intensity map in gray scale, as shown in (a). In (b) the FA is coded in the intensity values and the main diffusion direction is used for color coding. This allows a more detailed investigation of the diffusion. 33

4.6. The importance of color coding is illustrated on an enlargement of the centers of the images in Fig.4.5. The transition, for example, of the green and blue fibers in the center cannot be distinguished from the gray scale image. Some of these regions that are not distinguishable without color-coding are indicated with white arrows. 33

4.7. Comparison: Lamé ellipsoid vs. Reynolds tensor glyph 34

4.8. An example for the tensor visualization of the diffusion with lamé ellipsoids. For better orientation in the data set the intensity of the ellipsoid glyphs is coded according to the corresponding FA values and colored according to the orientation of their main axis. 35

4.9. Examples for spherical harmonics 36

4.10. The different orders of SHD are illustrated here. L and M corresponds to the spherical harmonic basis Y_M^L. The degree of the decompotition L indicates the underlying voxel fiber structure as indicated on the right. Odd degrees of the decomposition are assumed contain only artifacts. This graphic is taken from [32]. 37

4.11. The influence of the odd order tensor on the PDF is illustrated. 41

4.12. An example for the two kinds of HOT glyph for a pair of orthogonally crossing fibers. The HOTs were estimated from simulated data sets without noise and an force-minimizing encoding scheme [50] with 81 directions. (b) shows a cross-sectional cut through the synthetic phantom evaluated here (image adopted from [57]). The position of the evaluated voxel is indicated by the stippled line. 43

4.13. A comparison of the diffusion glyphs of the two presented HOT models for a splitting fiber. The HOTs were estimated from simulated data sets without noise and an force-minimizing encoding scheme [50] with 21 directions. (b) shows a cross-sectional cut through the synthetic phantom used to simulate the data evaluated here (image adopted from [57]). The position of the evaluated voxel is indicated by a stippled square. 44

List of Figures

4.14. A comparison of the diffusion glyphs. The lines give the extrema of the corresponding reconstructed PDF, which correspond to dominating diffusion directions. In (a) the input glyph is given. Below the evaluation with the single HOT (b) and the HOT hierarchy (c) are given with an increasing number of encoding directions from left to right ($N_e = 21, 30, 46, 81, 126$). The evaluations were performed on simulated data sets with SNR 20 and an force-minimizing encoding scheme [50]. . . . 45

5.1. This figure shows some examples for the triangulation of the regular icosahedron as means for mesh refinement. 47

5.2. Examples for the refinement of the icosahedral mesh. The dots give the position of the vertices of the refinement. 48

5.3. The points show the 126 encoding directions over the sphere that correspond to half the vertices of a refined icosahedron. 49

5.4. The points illustrate the distribution of the 126 encoding directions over the sphere as result of the analytical GES generation algorithms. 50

5.5. An example for the repulsion between the points on the sphere. 51

5.6. An example for an force minimizing direction sets with 126 directions. . 52

5.7. An example for a Cond GES with 126 directions. 52

6.1. The mean condition number evaluation results for the standard second order tensor estimation. The bar for Ana1 with $N_e = 15$ was interrupted to allow the discrimination of the small differences in the condition number for the better performing GES. 58

6.2. A more detailed look at the condition number evaluation results for the standard second order tensor estimation previously presented in Fig.6.1. The error bars in this figure give the minimal and maximal condition number encountered in all evaluated rotations. The length of these error bars gives the span of values for the corresponding condition number. Here, the bars for the Ana1 evaluations with N_e = 15, 16, 21, and 30 are omitted to enhance the relatively small differences of the better performing GES. 59

6.3. The mean condition number over all evaluated rotations for the HOT hierarchy. The value for Cond21 is very high and interrupted in this graph to show the small differences of the better performing GES more clearly. 62

6.4. A more detailed comparison of the mean condition number for the HOT hierarchy estimation with the best performing GES is given. In addition to the mean condition number the span of values for the rotational dependent condition numbers is given in the error-bars whose ends correspond to the minimal and maximal condition number over all evaluated rotations. The Y-axis starts at 470000 and is interrupted at 555000 to enhance the differences between the GES. 63

List of Figures

6.5. The mean rotationally dependent condition number for the single HOT model estimation. The comparatively high condition numbers for Cond and Ana1 with $N_e = 15-30$ as well as ForceSingle, and Ana2 with $N_e = 15 - 21$ are omitted in this graph to allow the distinction of relatively small differences in the better performing GES. 64

6.6. A more detailed comparison of the best performing GES for the single HOT estimation is given. The bars corresponding to GES with relatively high condition numbers are omitted here to enhance the differences of the GES with lower condition number. To improve the comparability the span of values for the rotationally dependent condition numbers is given in the error-bars which indicate the minimal and maximal condition number over all evaluated rotations. 65

6.7. The distribution of the diffusion encoding directions for the different GES families with $N_e = 126$. The blue dots represent the original directions and the red ones their inversion. 66

6.8. The clustering pairs in the ForceSingle GES (gradient directions (in blue) and their inversions (in red)). The direction sets were taken from the homepage of Robert Womersley (http://web.maths.unsw.edu.au/ rsw/sphere/). 67

6.9. The histogram of the angular distribution for GESs with $N_e = 81$ for each creation method. 68

6.10. The electrostatic energy histograms for the GES directions and their inversions. 70

6.11. Details from the electrostatic energy histograms in Fig.6.10 for the GES directions and their inversions. 71

6.12. The energy histograms of the best performing GESs are directly compared. 73

6.13. The two input tensor used in the simulation (each viewed in YZ and XZ plane). 74

6.14. The evaluation results for a tensor with one dominating eigenvalue (cigar-shaped tensor). The analytical and ForceSingle GESs require larger N_e, and can therefore not be used for the estimation with $N_e = 6$. 77

6.15. The evaluation results for a tensor with two equally large eigenvalues (oblate tensor). The analytical and ForceSingle GES cannot be used to estimate the second order tensor with $N_e = 6$. 78

6.16. The evaluation of the accuracy of the signal representation of the second order tensor with 21 directions. 81

6.17. The evaluation of the accuracy of the signal representation of the HOT hierarchy model with 21 directions. 81

6.18. The evaluation of the accuracy of the signal representation of the single HOT model with 21 directions. 82

6.19. The signal accuracy for ForcePairs GESs with increasing N_e. 84

6.20. The ADC glyph corresponding to the different tensor model derived signals for Icosa81 without noise in XY-plane. 85

List of Figures

6.21. The evaluation of the accuracy of the signal representation of the single HOT model with 21 directions and SNR 20. 86
6.22. The evaluation of the accuracy of the signal representation of the second order tensor with 21 directions and SNR 20. 86
6.23. The evaluation of the accuracy of the signal representation of the HOT hierarchy model with 21 directions and SNR 20. 87
6.24. The signal accuracy for ForcePairs GESs with increasing N_e on noisy data. 88

7.1. The thick dark arrow represents the fiber that is to be reconstructed. The tract reconstructed with steps of equal size (in red) deviates from the fiber that is to be reconstructed. It can be seen that the reconstruction on a continuous vector field (thin black arrows) track the path of the fiber more accurately. The graphic was adapted from [68]. 95
7.2. The effect of tensor averaging is illustrated by two crossing fibers. On the fibers the diffusion glyphs are cigar shaped. In the intersection of the fiber pathways the shape gets more spherical, that is less anisotropic. The fiber running from left to right (red) is slightly dominating the top-down (green) pathway. This plot was generated with the TensorViewer of the MedInria software package [29]. 96
7.3. Tract reconstruction with 'brute force' (a) and filtering of the results with one (b) or multiple ROIs (c). The positions of the ROIs are marked on an axial FA slice in (d). 96
7.4. Illustration of the front propagation with the fast-marching technique. The front propagation depends on the normal of the front ($n(\mathbf{r})$) and the principal eigenvectors in the individual voxels (lines through the points). This figures are adapted from [78]. 97
7.5. The results of a probabilistic tracking method (overlayed on a FA map), generated with the FSL/FDT [31] software package. 100

8.1. The flattening of the sides of the initial peak will enlarge the ROI that is used in tracking. This is illustrated in the comparison of an Dirac-like peak (left) with a Gaussian peak (right). In the lower row of images the size of the projected ROI is illustrated. The size of the ROI corresponding to the Gaussian peak corresponds to the outermost ring in (d). The size of the ROI in (c) is exactly one voxel. 103
8.2. The approximation of the flux with finite differences is illustrated. . . . 106
8.3. A comparison of the TOAs of the fast marching method (a) and the DSBT method (b). The DSBT method covers more data points in one time step. The steps in the TOA are wider than in the one created by the fast-marching technique. 107
8.4. The concentration (colored curves) may underrun a constant threshold (stipled line) if several time steps are evaluated. 107

List of Figures

8.5. The detection of the diffusion fronts illustrated on the example of isotropic diffusion in 2D. The main difference between the methods is the size of the flooded region for the individual time steps.   109
8.6. The method of histogram classification is illustrated here. The classification threshold is chosen to guarantee a predefined minimal number of points to be flooded in each time step.   109
8.7. The gradient descend reconstructs a tract from the outermost front (dark red) in the TOA map toward the simulation origin (dark blue). The different time stamps in the TOA map are illustrated as colored bars. . . .   110
8.8. The increase in possible tracts for each simulation time step is illustrated here.   111
8.9. The concentration values of all points flooded the first time in a time step (blue striped region, between stippled lines) is used to compute the concentration values. The region between the red lines was previously flooded and is therefore not considered in this step.   111
8.10. The simulation and therefore the TOA map will bleed into the background if diffusivity outside of the fiber is not ideally zero (a). The background can be filtered by thresholding the anisotropy, as shown in (b). .   112
8.11. The simulated diffusion in (a) is bleeding into the background and from there again into the spiral. (b) shows that the bleeding in the background can be masked by anisotropy thresholding but on reentering the tract it will cause problems for the tracking algorithm. The region where the diffusion is entering the inner winding of the spiral through the background is indicated with an arrow in each image.   113
8.12. An illustration of the straight line bridging of the gap between the boundary of the initial peak (dark blue on the right) and the original ROI (white dot). (a) shows the TOA map of a simple fiber example. This map is discretized to the data grid in (b). In (c) two exemplary reconstructed tracts are plotted in gray over the TOA map. In (d) the trackts are connected to the original ROI with a straight line.   114
8.13. The subgrid is a small region in the data volume.   115
8.14. This graphic illustrates the successive evaluation of the diffusion simulation on small subregions. The simulation results are depicted as black lines that represent the outermost diffusion front. The black dot marks the simulation origin. The red line stands for the reconstructed tract piece. From the second simulation onward, the number of points, that can be part of a valid tract, are reduced because of the smoothness criteria. The reduction of the points is illustrated with the dotted black cutting plane. The arrows attached to this plane indicate, which part of the diffusion front will be considered in the evaluation.   116
8.15. To avoid effects of the boundary condition a border is introduced to the subgrid.   117

List of Figures

8.16. When the simulated diffusion is isotropic, the fiber will be reconstructed as straight line until a boundary is reached. The effect is most prominent in curving fibers (b). 118

8.17. Merger of the path of two tracts that are similar ($d < C_s$). 121

8.18. The global smoothness depends on the angle α between the average tract directions d_i. The first tract reconstructs a path between pp_seed and p_seed. The second one starts in p_seed and ends in seed. 122

8.19. An overview over the class structure of the implementation. 126

8.20. A flow chart of the algorithm. The steps are color and shape coded, according to the class they belong to: green - rectangular corresponds to the main DSBT method; red - round rectangles correspond to BuildMapSG2; dark red - oval, corresponds to the SG2 simulation and blue - stretched circle corresponds to GradientDescendOnFront. The small red signs (F) mark the path taken when the loop condition or the condition in the corresponding diamond is false, the green signs (T) mark paths for true conditions. 127

8.21. The tracking results for a simulated branching fiber. 128

8.22. The influence of the similarity termination criterion on the reconstruction. 129

8.23. The influence of the subvoxel size on the results illustrated on a simulated branching fiber. 130

8.24. The tracking results for two orthogonally crossing fibers. 131

8.25. The tracking results for a straight crossing fibers. 132

8.26. A detailed view of the tensors in the region of crossing. This plot was generated with the TensorViewer of the MedInria software package [29]. 132

8.27. Curved crossing and kissing fibers have an ambiguous tensor profile. The first column gives the position of the detailed plots in the second column in the data set. The plots were created with the Camino software [21]. . 134

8.28. The tracking results for curved crossing fibers. 134

8.29. The tracking results for a kissing set of fibers. 135

8.30. The tracking results for a spiraling fiber. 135

8.31. The tensor glyphs of the inner end of the spiral tract show a random orientation that prevents further reconstruction. This plot was generated with the TensorViewer of the MedInria software package [29]. 136

8.32. The interpolations needed for the more advanced diffusion simulation are illustrated here in a 2D scheme for one exemplary gradient direction **d**. The flux (8.9) is estimated for the point in the center, marked with a yellow star. The points on the fiber are given in blue, the ones on the background in orange. The 2D diffusion ellipsoid, corresponding to the second order diffusion tensor, illustrates the corresponding (Gaussian) diffusion profiles. The ADCs, corresponding to direction **d** (ADC_f), and −**d** (ADC_b) are illustrated with red arrows. They are computed by linear interpolation, first between neighboring data points along the green lines, and then along the gray dotted line. 138

F. List of Tables

6.1. ν is evaluated for different GES with $N_e = 46$. 57
6.2. The mean condition numbers for the GES evaluation of the single HOT model of order 6. 60
6.3. The condition number results for the Icosa GES evaluation the HOT hierarchy of order four. 61
6.4. The condition number results for the Icosa GES evaluating the single HOT model of order four. 61
6.5. Number of point pairs with an energy value greater four. 69
6.6. The tensor estimation results for a cigar shaped tensor for the best performing GESs with $N_e = 30$. 79
6.7. The tensor estimation results for an oblate shaped tensor for the best performing GESs with $N_e = 30$. 79
6.8. Maximum of the $\bar{\epsilon}$ over all rotations. 82
6.9. Mean and standard deviation of the $\bar{\epsilon}$ over all rotations. 83
6.10. Maximum of the mean error over all rotations on noisy data. 86
6.11. Mean and standard deviation of $\bar{\epsilon}$ over all rotations on noisy data. . . . 87

A.1. The mean condition number evaluated for the second order tensor. . . . 144
A.2. The condition number evaluated for the second order tensor. 144
A.3. The condition number evaluated for the second order tensor (continued). 145
A.4. The condition number evaluated for the fourth order single HOT model. 145
A.5. The condition number evaluated for the fourth order single HOT model. 146
A.6. The condition number evaluated for the fourth order HOT hierarchy (even order estimation matrix). 146
A.7. The condition number evaluated for the fourth order HOT hierarchy (continued). 146
A.8. The condition number evaluated for the fourth order HOT hierarchy (continued). 146
A.9. The condition number evaluated for the sixth order single HOT model. . 147
A.10. The condition number evaluated for the sixth order single HOT model (continued). 147
A.11. The condition number evaluated for the sixth order HOT hierarchy (even order estimation matrix). 147
A.12. The condition number evaluated for the sixth order HOT hierarchy (continued). 147

List of Tables

A.13. The condition number evaluated for the sixth order HOT hierarchy (continued). 147
A.14. The condition number evaluated for the eighth order single HOT model. 148
A.15. The condition number evaluated for the eighth order single HOT model (continued). 148
A.16. The condition number evaluated for the eighth order single HOT model. 148

Abbreviations

$\bar{D}$ mean diffusivity

λ_i eigenvalue with index i

N_e number of encoding directions

T_1 imaging contrast, depending on longitudinal magnetization

T_2/T_2^* imaging contrast, depending on dephasing of transversal magnetization.

tr tensor trace

B   estimation matrix

Y   vector containing the logarithm of the divisions of diffusion weighted and unweighted signals

ADC   apparent diffusion coefficient

DSBT   diffusion simulation based tracking

DTI   diffusion tensor imaging

DWI   diffusion weighted imaging

EPI   echo planar imaging

FA   fractional anisotropy

FV   finite volumes

GES   gradient encoding scheme

GM   (brain) gray matter

HARDI   higher angular resolution diffusion imaging

HOT   higher order tensor

MRI   magnetic resonance imaging

Abbreviations

PDE	partial differential equation
PDF	probability density function
PVE	partial volume effect
QSI	**q**-space imaging
RA	relative anisotropy
RF	radio frequency
ROI	region of interest
SLT	streamline tracking
SNR	signal to noise ration
TE	echo time, amount of time between excitation and echo generation
TOA	time of arrival
TR	repetition time, amount of time that passes between two excitations
WM	(brain) white matter

Original Publications

[Mang05] Mang, S., Gembris, D. and Männer, R. Rekonstruktion von neuronalen Trajektorien mittels Time-of-Arrival-Maps. *Workshop Bildverarbeitung für die Medizin* (2005), 267-271.

[Mang05a] Mang, S., Gembris, D. and Männer, R. Reconstruction of neuronal fiber tracts using Time-of-Arrival-Maps. *ISMRM workshop on methods for quantitative diffusion MRI of human brain* (2005)

[Mang05b] Mang, S., Gembris, D. and Männer, R. Tracking white matter fibers using time of arrival maps. *ESMRMB* (2005)

[Mang06] Mang, S., Kang, N., Zhang, J., Carlson, E. S. and Gembris, D. Current state of diffusion simulation based tractography. *ISMRM 14th annual meeting* (2006) 2737

[Mang07] Mang, S., Gembris, D. and Männer, R. Evaluation of the higher order tensor estimation quality for established gradient encoding schemes. *Joint Annual Meeting ISMRM-ESMRMB* (2007) 3165

[Mang07a] Mang, S., Gembris, D. and Männer, R. Comparison of the tensor estimation quality for icosahedral gradient encoding schemes. *Joint Annual Meeting ISMRM-ESMRMB* (2007) 5158

[Liu07] Liu, C., Mang, C., Moseley, M. E. In Vivo Generalized Diffusion Tensor Imaging and Higher Order Diffusion Contrasts. *SNDS bi-national workshop on: MRI of brain connectivity and microstructure: Measurement and Validation* (2007)

[Gembris07a] Gembris, D., Mang, S. and Männer, R. Diffusion Simulation Based Tractography (DST): Current Results and Outlook. *SNDS bi-national workshop on: MRI of brain connectivity and microstructure: Measurement and Validation* (2007)

[Gembris07b] Gembris, D., Logashenko, D., Mang, S., Wittum, G., and Männer, R. Superresolution Approach for Diffusion Tensor Imaging based on Diffusion Modeling*SNDS bi-national workshop on: MRI of brain connectivity and microstructure: Measurement and Validation* (2007)

F. Original Publications

[Mang08] Mang S., Logashenko D., Gembris D., Wittum G., and Männer R. Extending Diffusion Simulation Based Tractography (DSBT) To Other Diffusion Models. *Annual Meeting ISMRM* (2008) submitted

Bibliography

[1] AG TECHNISCHE SIMULATION DER UNIVERSITÄT HEIDELBERG. *SG2*. http://sourceforge.net/projects/sg2/, 2007.

[2] ALEXANDER, A. L., HASAN, K. M., LAZAR, M., TSURUDA, J. S., AND PARKER, D. L. Analysis of Partial Volume Effects in Diffusion-Tensor MRI. *Magnetic Resonance In Medicine 45*, 5 (2001), 770–780.

[3] ALEXANDER, D. C., BARKER, G. J., AND ARRIDGE, S. R. Detection and Modeling of Non-Gaussian Apparent Diffusion Coefficient Profiles in Human Brain Data. *Magnetic Resonance In Medicine 48*, 2 (2002), 331–340.

[4] ASSAF, Y., FREIDLIN, R. Z., ROHDE, G. K., AND BASSER, P. J. New Modeling and Experimental Framework to Characterize Hindered and Restricted Water Diffusion in Brain White Matter. *Magnetic Resonance In Medicine 52*, 5 (2004), 965–978.

[5] BARRETT, R., BERRY, M., CHAN, T. F., DEMMEL, J., DONATO, J., DONGARRA, J., EIJKHOUT, V., POZO, R., ROMINE, C., AND VAN DER VORST, H. *Templates for the solution of linear systems: building blocks for iterative methods*. SIAM, Philadelphia, PA, 1993.

[6] BASSER, P. J. Inferring microstructural features and physiological state of tissues from diffusion-weighted images. *NMR In Biomedicine 8* (1995), 333–344.

[7] BASSER, P. J. Relationships Between Diffusion Tensor and q-Space MRI. *Magnetic Resonance In Medicine 47* (2002), 392–397.

[8] BASSER, P. J., PAJEVIC, S., PIERPAOLI, C., DUDA, J., AND ALDROUBI, A. In Vivo Fiber Tractography Using DT-MRI Data. *Magnetic Resonance IMAging 44*, 4 (2000), 625–632.

[9] BASSER, P. J., AND PIERPAOLI, C. A Simplified Method to Measure the Diffusion Tensor from Seven MR Images. *Magnetic Resonance In Medicine 39* (1998), 928–934.

[10] BATCHELOR, P. G., ATKINSON, D., HILL, D. L. G., CALAMANTE, F., AND CONNELLY, A. Anisotropic Noise Propagation in Diffusion Tensor MRI Sampling Schemes. *Magnetic Resonance In Medicine 49*, 6 (2003), 1143–1151.

F. Bibliography

[11] BATCHELOR, P. G., HILL, D. L. G., CALAMANTE, F., AND ATKINSON, D. Study of Connectivity in the Brain Using the Full Diffusion Tensor from MRI. In *IPMI '01: Proceedings of the 17th International Conference on Information Processing in Medical Imaging* (London, UK, 2001), Lecture Notes in Computer Science, Springer, pp. 121–133.

[12] BEAULIEU, C. The basis of anisotropic water diffusion in the nervous system - a technical review. *NMR In Biomedicine 15*, 7-8 (2002), 435–455.

[13] BEHRENS, T. E. J., WOOLRICH, M. W., JENKINSON, M., JOHANSEN-BERG, H., NUNES, R. G., CLARE, S., MATTHEWS, P. M., BRANDY, J. M., AND SMITH, S. M. Characterization and Propagation of Uncertainty in Diffusion-Weighted MR Imaging. *Magnetic Resonance In Medicine 50*, 5 (2003), 1077–1088.

[14] BROWN, M. A., AND SEMELKA, R. C. *MRI - BASIC PRINCIPLES AND APPLICATIONS, THIRD EDITION*. John Wiley and Sons, Inc., 2003.

[15] BUERGEL, U., SCHORMANN, T., SCHLEICHER, A., AND ZILLES, K. Mapping of Histologically Identified Long Fiber Tracts in Human Cerebral Hemispheres to the MRI Volume of a Referance Brain: Position and Spatial Variability of Optic Radiation. *Neuroimage 10* (1999), 489–499.

[16] CALLAGHAN, P. T. *Principles of Nuclear Magnetic Resonance Microscopy*. Oxford University Press, 1993.

[17] CALLAGHAN, P. T., COY, A., MACGOWAN, D., PACKER, K. J., AND ZELAYA, F. O. Diffraction-like effects in NMR diffusion studies of fluids in porous solids. *Nature 351* (1991), 467–469.

[18] CAMPBELL, J. S. W., SIDDIQI, K., AND PIKE, G. B. White Matter Fibre Tractography and Scalar Connectivity Assessment Using Fiber Orientation Likelihood Distribution. In *2004 IEEE Computer Society Conference on Computer Vision and Pattern Recognition – CVPR 2004* (2004), IEEE Computer Society.

[19] COMSOL. *FEMLAB*. http://www.femlab.de/, 2005.

[20] CONTURO, T. E., LORI, N. F., CULL, T. S., AKBUDAK, E., SNYDER, A. Z., SHIMONY, J. S., MCKINSTRY, R. C., BURTON, H., AND RAICHLE, M. E. Tracking neuronal fiber pathways in the living human brain. *Proceedings of The National Academy Of Sciences Of The United States Of America 96*, 18 (1999), 10422–10427.

[21] COOK, P. A., BAI, Y., NEDJATI-GILANI, S., SEUNARINE, M., HALL, M. G., PARKER, G. J., AND ALEXANDER, D. C. Camino: Open-source diffusion-mri reconstruction and processing. In *14th ISMRM Meeting 2006* (2006), p. 2759.

[22] CRANK, J. *The Mathematics of Diffusion*. Oxford University Press, 1975.

[23] CUI, J., AND FREEDEN, W. Equidistribution on the sphere. *SIAM J. Sci: Comput. 18* (1997), 595–609.

[24] DELMARCELLE, T., AND HESSELINK, L. Visualizing second-order tensor fields with hyperstream lines. *IEEE Computer Graphics and Applications 13*, 4 (1993), 25–33.

[25] DEONI, S. C. L., AND JONES, D. K. Generation of a common diffusion tensor imaging dataset. In *Proceedings of the ISMRM Workshop on "Methods for Quantitative Diffusion MRI of Human Brain"* (2005).

[26] DESCOTEAUX, M., ANGELINO, E., FITZGIBBONS, S., AND DERICHE, R. Apparent diffusion coefficients from high angular resolution diffusion imaging: estimation and applications. *Magnetic Resonance In Medicine 56*, 2 (Aug 2006), 395–410.

[27] EFRON, B. Bootstrap methods: another look at the jackknife. *The Annals of Statistics 7* (1979), 1–16.

[28] EHRICKE, H.-H., KLOSE, U., AND GRODD, W. Visualizing MR diffusion tensor fields by dynamic fiber tracking and probability mapping. *IEEE Computer Graphics and Applications* (2006).

[29] FILLARD, P., SOUPLET, J.-C., AND TOUSSAINT, N. *Medical Image Navigation and Research Tool by INRIA (MedINRIA)*. INRIA Sophia Antipolis - Research Project ASCLEPIOS, 2007.

[30] FLIEGE, J., AND MAIER, U. The distribution of points on the sphere and corresponding cubature formulae. *IMA Journal of Numerical Analysis 19*, 2 (1999), 317–334.

[31] FMRIB ANALYSIS GROUP. *FSL*. Oxford University, UK, 2007.

[32] FRANK, L. R. Characterization of Anisotropy in High Angular Resolution Diffusion-Weighted MRI. *Magnetic Resonance In Medicine 47* (2002), 1083–1099.

[33] GEMBRIS, D. *Rekonstruktion Neuronaler Konnektivität Mittels Kernmagnetischer Resonanz*. PhD thesis, University of Dortmund, 2001.

[34] GLOVER, G. H. Simple analytic spiral k-space algorithm. *Magnetic Resonance In Medicine 42*, 2 (1999), 412–415.

[35] GROSSMANN, C., AND ROOS, H.-G. *Numerik partieller Differentialgleichungen*. Teubner, Stuttgart, 1994.

F. Bibliography

[36] HAACKE, E. M., BROWN, R. W., THOMPSON, M. R., AND VENKATESAN, R. *Magnetic Resonance Imaging - Physical Principles ans Sequence Design.* Wiley-Liss, 1999.

[37] HACKBUSCH, W. *Iterative Solution of Large Sparse Systems of Equations.* Springer, New-York, 1994.

[38] HAHN, E. L. Spin echoes. *Physical Review 80*, 4 (Nov 1950), 580–594.

[39] HAHN, E. L., AND MAXWELL, D. E. Spin echo measurements of nuclear spin coupling in molecules. *Physical Review 88*, 5 (Dec 1952), 1070–1084.

[40] HASAN, K. M., ALEXANDER, A. L., AND NARAYANA, P. A. Does fractional anisotropy have better noise immunity characteristics than relative anisotropy in diffusion tensor MRI? An analytical approach. *Magnetic Resonance In Medicine 51* (2004), 413–417.

[41] HASAN, K. M., AND NARAYANA, P. A. Computation of the fractional anisotropy and mean diffusivity maps without tensor decoding and diagonalization: Theoretical analysis and validation. *Magnetic Resonance In Medicine 50*, 3 (Sep 2003), 589–598.

[42] HASAN, K. M., PARKER, D. L., AND ALEXANDER, A. L. Comparison of Gradient Encoding Schemes for Diffusion-Tensor MRI. *Journal of magnetic resonance imaging : JMRI. 13* (2001), 769–780.

[43] HASHASH, Y. M. A., YAO, J. I.-C., AND WOTRING, D. C. Glyph and hyperstreamline representation of stress and strain tensor and material constitutive response. *International Journal for Numerical and Analytical Methods in Geomechanics 27* (2003), 603–626.

[44] JACKOWSKI, M., KAO, C. Y., QIU, M., CONSTABLE, R. T., AND STAIB, L. H. Estimation of Anatomical Connectivity by Anisotropic Front Propagation and Diffusion Tensor Imaging. In *Medical Image Computing and Computer-Assisted Intervention – MICCAI 2004* (2004), C. Barillot, D. R. Haynor, and P. Hellier, Eds., vol. 3217 of *Lecture Notes in Computer Science*, Springer, pp. 663–670.

[45] JONES, D. K. Determining and visualizing uncertainty in estimates of fiber orientation from diffusion tensor MRI. *Magnetic Resonance In Medicine 49*, 1 (Jan 2003), 7–12.

[46] JONES, D. K. When is a DT-MRI sampling scheme truly isotropic? In *Annual Meeting of the ISMRM* (2003).

[47] JONES, D. K. The effect of gradient sampling schemes on measures derived from diffusion tensor MRI: a Monte Carlo study. *Magnetic Resonance In Medicine 51*, 4 (Apr 2004), 807–815.

[48] JONES, D. K., AND BASSER, P. J. "Squashing peanuts and smashing pumpkins": how noise distorts diffusion-weighted MR data. *Magnetic Resonance In Medicine 52*, 5 (Nov 2004), 979–993.

[49] JONES, D. K., HORSFIELD, M. A., AND SIMMONS, A. Optimal Strategies for Measureing Diffusion in Anisotropic Systems by Magnetic Resonance Imaging. *Magnetic Resonance In Medicine 42*, 3 (1999), 515–525.

[50] JONES, D. K., SIMMONS, A., WILLIAMS, S. C., AND HORSFIELD, M. A. Non-invasive assessment of axonal fiber connectivity in the human brain via diffusion tensor MRI. *Magnetic Resonance In Medicine 42*, 1 (Jul 1999), 37–41.

[51] KANG, N., ZHANG, J., CARLSON, E. S., AND GEMBRIS, D. White Matter Fiber Tractography via Anisotropic Diffusion Simulation in the Human Brain. *IEEE Transactions on Medical Imaging 24*, 9 (2005), 1127–1137.

[52] KINGSLEY, P. B. Introduction to diffusion tensor imaging mathematics: Part ii. tensor calculations, noise, simulations and optimization. *Concepts in Magnetic Resonance Part A 28*, 2 (2006), 123–154.

[53] KINGSLEY, P. B. Introduction to diffusion tensor imaging mathematics: Part iii. tensor calculation, noise, simulations, and optimization. *Concepts in Magnetic Resonance Part A 28A*, 2 (2006), 155–179.

[54] KREHER, B. W., SCHNEIDER, J. F., MADER, I., MARTIN, E., HENNIG, J., AND IL'YASOV, K. A. Multitensor approach for analysis and tracking of complex fiber configurations. *Magnetic Resonance In Medicine 54*, 5 (Nov 2005), 1216–1225.

[55] KROENKE, C. D., BRETTHORST, G. L., INDER, T. E., AND NEIL, J. J. Modeling water diffusion anisotropy within fixed newborn primate brain using Bayesian probability theory. *Magnetic Resonance In Medicine 55*, 1 (Jan 2006), 187–197.

[56] LENGLET, C., DERICHE, R., AND FAUGERAS, O. Inferring White Matter Geometry from Diffusion Tensor MRI: Application to Connectivity Mapping. In *Proceedings of the 8th European Conference on Computer Vision* (2004), T. Pajdla and J. Matas, Eds., Springer, pp. 127–140.

[57] LIU, C., BAMMER, R., ACAR, B., AND MOSELEY, M. E. Characterizing non-Gaussian diffusion by using generalized diffusion tensors. *Magnetic Resonance In Medicine 51*, 5 (May 2004), 924–937.

[58] LIU, C., BAMMER, R., AND MOSELEY, M. E. Generalized Diffusion Tensor Imaging (GDTI): A Method for Characterizing and Imaging Diffusion Anisotropy Caused by Non-Gaussian Diffusion. *Israel Journal of Chemistry 43* (2003), 145–154.

F. Bibliography

[59] LIU, C., BAMMER, R., AND MOSELEY, M. E. Limitations of Apparent Diffusion Coefficient-Based Models in Characterizing Non-Gaussian Diffusion. *Magnetic Resonance In Medicine 54* (2005), 419–428.

[60] LIU, C., MOSELEY, M. E., AND BAMMER, R. Simultaneous phase correction and sense reconstruction for navigated multi-shot dwi with non-cartesian k-space sampling. *Magnetic Resonance in Medicine 54*, 6 (2005), 1412–1422.

[61] LORI, N. F., AKBUDAK, E., SHIMONY, J. S., CULL, T. S., SNYDER, A. Z., GUILLORY, R. K., AND CONTURO, T. E. Diffusion tensor fiber tracking of human brain connectivity: aquisition methods, reliability analysis and biological results. *NMR In Biomedicine 15*, 7-8 (2002), 492–515.

[62] MANSFIELD, P., COXON, R., AND HYKIN, J. Echo-volumar imaging (EVI) of the brain at 3.0 T: first normal volunteer and functional imaging results. *Journal of Computer Assisted Tomography 19*, 6 (1995), 847–852.

[63] MATTIELLO, J., BASSER, P. J., AND BIHAN, D. L. The b Matrix in Diffusion Tensor Echo-Planar Imaging. *Magnetic Resonance In Medicine 37* (1997), 292–300.

[64] MCCULLAGH, P. *Tensor Methods in Statistics*. Chapman and Hall, 1987.

[65] MITRA, P. P., AND HALPERIN, B. I. Effects of Finite Gradient-Pulse Widths in Pulsed-Field-Gradient Diffusion Measurements. *Journal of Magnetic Resonance, Series A 113* (1995), 94–101.

[66] MOORE, J. G., SCHORN, S. A., AND MOORE, J. Methods of classical mechanics applied in turbulence stresses in a tip leakage vortex. In *AMSE: 11th International Gas Turbine and Aeroengine Congress & Exposition, Houston, Texas* (1995).

[67] MORI, S. *Introduction to Diffusion Tensor Imaging*. Elsevier, 2007.

[68] MORI, S., CRAIN, B. J., CHACKO, V. P., AND VAN ZIJL, P. C. M. Three-Dimensional Tracking of Axonal Projections in the Brain by Magnetic Resonance Imaging. *Annals of Neurology 45*, 2 (1999), 265–269.

[69] MORI, S., AND VAN ZIJL, P. C. M. Fiber tracking: principles and strategies - a technical review. *NMR In Biomedicine 15* (2002), 468–480.

[70] MUTHUPALLAI, R., C. A. HOLDER, A. W. S., AND DIXON, W. T. Navigator aided multishot EPI diffusion images of brain with complete orientation and anisotropy information. In *7th Annual Meeting of ISMRM* (Philadelphia, 1999), vol. 27, p. 1825.

[71] NELSON, E. *Dynamical theories of Brownian Motion*. Princeton University Press, 1967.

[72] NILSSON, M., AND ROSQUIST, H. q-space diffusion MRI: Sequence development and phantom design. Master's thesis, Lund University, 2006.

[73] OEZARSLAN, E., AND MARECI, T. H. Generalized Diffusion Tensor Imaging and Analytical Relationships Between Diffusion Tensor Imaging and High Angular Resolution Diffusion Imaging. *Magnetic Resonance In Medicine 50* (2003), 955–965.

[74] OEZARSLAN, E., VEMURI, B. C., AND MARECI, T. H. Generalized Scalar Measures for Diffusion MRI Using Trace, Variance and Entropy. *Magnetic Resonance In Medicine 53* (2005), 866–876.

[75] PAPADAKIS, N. G., XING, D., HUANG, C. L., HALL, L. D., AND CARPENTER, T. A. A comparative study of acquisition schemes for diffusion tensor imaging using MRI. *Journal of Magnetic Resonance 137*, 1 (Mar 1999), 67–82.

[76] PAPADAKIS, N. G., XING, D., HUANG, C. L.-H., HALL, L. D., AND CARPENTER, T. A. A Comparative Study of Acquisition Schemes for Diffusion Tensor Imaging Using MRI. *Journal of Magnetic Resonance 137*, 1 (1999), 67–82.

[77] PARKER, G. J. M., HAROON, H. A., AND WHEELER-KINGSHOTT, C. A. A Framework for a Streamline-Based Probabilistic Index of Connectivity (PICo) Using a Structural Interpretation of MRI Diffusion Measurements. *Magnetic Resonance In Medicine 18* (2003), 242–254.

[78] PARKER, G. J. M., WHEELER-KINGSHOTT, C. A. M., AND BARKER, G. J. Distributed Anatomical Brain Connectivity Derived from Diffusion Tensor Imaging. In *Information Processing in Medical Imaging 17th International Conference* (2001), pp. 106–120.

[79] PARKER, G. J. M., WHEELER-KINGSHOTT, C. A. M., AND BARKER, G. J. Estimating Distributed Anatomical Connectivity Using Fast Marching Methods and Diffusion Tensor Imaging. *IEEE Transactions on Medical Imaging 21*, 5 (2002), 505–512.

[80] PENG, H., AND ARFANAKIS, K. Diffusion tensor encoding schemes optimized for white matter fibers with selected orientations. *Magnetic Resonance Imaging*, 25 (2007), 147–153.

[81] POONAWALLA, A. H., AND ZHOU, X. J. Analytical Error Propagation in Diffusion Anisotropy Calculations. *Journal of magnetic resonance imaging : JMRI. 19*, 4 (2004), 489–498.

[82] SCHÜNKE, M., SCHULTE, E., SCHUMACHER, U., VOLL, M., AND WESKER, K. *Prometheus, LernAtlas der Anatomie, Kopf und Neuroanatomie*. Thieme, 2006.

F. Bibliography

[83] SETHIAN, J. A. A fast marching level set method for monotonically advancing fronts. *Proceedings of The National Academy Of Sciences Of The United States Of America 93*, 4 (Feb 1996), 1591–1595.

[84] SKARE, S., HEHEHUS, M., MOSELEY, M. E., AND LI, T.-Q. Condition Number as a Measure of Noise Performance of Diffusion Tensor Data Acquisition Schemes with MRI. *Journal of Magnetic Resonance 147*, 2 (2000), 340–352.

[85] STAFF, E. B., AND KUIJLAARS, A. B. J. Distributing many points on a sphere. *Mathematical Intelligencer 19*, 1 (1997), 5–11.

[86] STEJSKAL, E. O., AND TANNER, J. E. Spin diffusion measurement: spin echoes in the presence of a time-dependent field gradient. *Journal of Chemical Physics 42* (1965), 288–292.

[87] STIELTJES, B., KAUFMANN, W. E., VAN ZIJL, P. C. M., FREDRICKSEN, K., PEARLSON, G. D., AND MORI, S. Diffusion Tensor Imaging and Axonal Tracking in the Human Brainstem. *Neuroimage 14* (2001), 723–735.

[88] TREFETHEN, L. N., AND DAVID BAU, I. *Numerical Linear Algebra*. SIAM, 1997.

[89] TREPEL, M. *Neuroanatomie - Struktur und Funktion*, 3. ed. Urban & Fischer, 2004.

[90] TUCH, D. S. *Diffusion MRI of Complex Tissue Structure*. PhD thesis, Harvard University-Massachusetts, Institute of Technology, 2002.

[91] TUCH, D. S., REESE, T. G., WIEGELL, M. R., MAKRIS, N., BELLIVEAU, J. W., AND WEDEEN, V. J. High angular resolution diffusion Imaging reveals intravoxel white matter fiber heterogeneity. *Magnetic Resonance In Medicine 48* (2002), 577–582.

[92] WEICKERT, J., AND HAGEN, H., Eds. *Visualization and processing of tensor fields*. Springer, 2006, ch. 1, pp. 3–13.

[93] WEISHAUPT, D., KOECHLI, V. D., AND MARINCEK, B. *Wie funktioniert MRI? - Eine Einführung in Physik und Funktionsweise der Magnetresonanzbildgebung*, 4 ed. Springer, 2003.

[94] WONG, S. T., AND ROOS, M. S. A strategy for sampling on a sphere applied to 3d selective rf pulse design. *Magnetic Resonance In Medicine 32*, 6 (Dec 1994), 778–784.

[95] ZHANG, S., DEMIRALP, C., AND LAIDLAW, D. Visualizing diffusion tensor MR images using streamtubes and streamsurfaces. *IEEE Transactions on Visualization and Computer Graphics 9*, 4 (Oct.-Dec. 2003), 454–462.

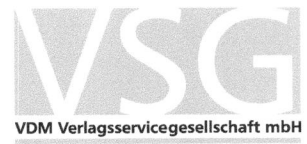

Die VDM Verlagsservicegesellschaft sucht für wissenschaftliche Verlage abgeschlossene und herausragende

Dissertationen, Habilitationen, Diplomarbeiten, Master Theses, Magisterarbeiten usw.

für die kostenlose Publikation als Fachbuch.

Sie verfügen über eine Arbeit, die hohen inhaltlichen und formalen Ansprüchen genügt, und haben Interesse an einer honorarvergüteten Publikation?

Dann senden Sie bitte erste Informationen über sich und Ihre Arbeit per Email an *info@vdm-vsg.de*.

Sie erhalten kurzfristig unser Feedback!

VDM Verlagsservicegesellschaft mbH
Dudweiler Landstr. 99   Telefon +49 681 3720 174
D - 66123 Saarbrücken   Fax   +49 681 3720 1749
www.vdm-vsg.de

Die VDM Verlagsservicegesellschaft mbH vertritt

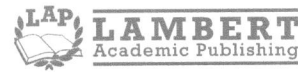
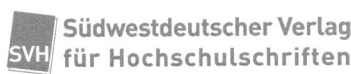

MIX
Papier aus verantwortungsvollen Quellen
Paper from responsible sources
FSC® C105338

Printed by Books on Demand GmbH, Norderstedt / Germany